Control Your ACID REFLUX, HEARTBURN & GERD:

A Doctor's Practical Guide that Works

Control Your ACID REFLUX, HEARTBURN & GERD:

A Doctor's Practical Guide that Works

Dr Prabhat Das
MD, PhD, FACP

Better Health with Dr Das Series

Disclaimer

This book is intended solely for educational and informational purposes. It is not meant to replace personal medical advice, diagnosis, or treatment. Although I am a licensed physician, reading this book does not establish a doctor–patient relationship. Each individual's health condition, medical history, and risk factors are unique. Any medical decision should be made in partnership with your own healthcare professional who understands your specific situation. Medical science is continually advancing. New research and updated guidelines may lead to changes in recommendations over time.

Hardcover ISBN: **978-1-971672-27-4**
Paperback ISBN: **978-1-971672-26-7**
eBook ISBN: **978-1-971672-25-0**

Typeset in font *Times New Roman* by *Indica Infomedia*, New Delhi, India
Printed in the United States of America

About the Author

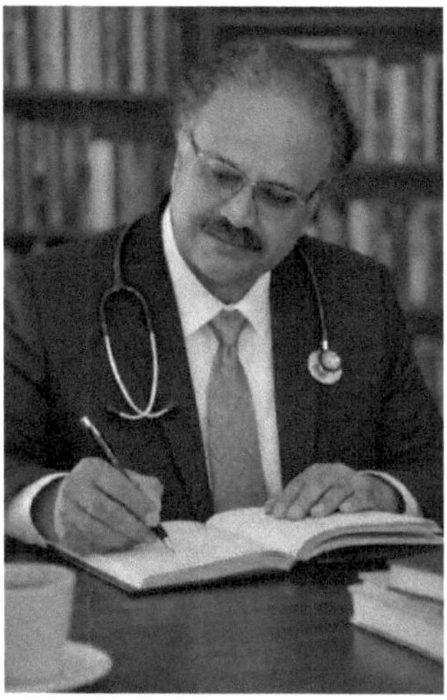

I am **Dr Prabhat Das**, MD, PhD, FACP. My journey in medicine began in India and, over the past thirty-five years, has continued in the United States, where I have had the privilege of caring for patients across a wide range of medical settings. I am trained in Internal Medicine, Pulmonary Diseases, and Critical Care. For me, medicine has never been just a profession. It has been a lifelong commitment shaped by learning, service, and a deep respect for the trust patients place in their physician.

Over the years, I have had the honor of caring for patients in many different situations. I have seen individuals in my office for routine concerns, treated urgent conditions in busy emergency rooms, managed serious illnesses in the hospital, and cared for critically ill patients in intensive care units. Each setting has taught me something valuable. Each patient has added to my understanding of what it truly means to care for another human being.

But one lesson has stood above all others. Medicine is not only about tests, diagnoses, or treatments. It is about people. It is about listening carefully, understanding fears that are often left unspoken, and guiding patients through uncertainty with clarity and compassion. Again and again, I have seen that what people want most is simple, trustworthy information. They want to understand what is happening in their bodies. They want to feel confident about the decisions they are making for their health and for their families.

These experiences have deeply shaped how I think about health, illness, prevention, and the human side of healing.

That is the reason behind the '**Better Health with Dr Das Series**'. Through these books, I hope to reach individuals I may never meet in person but who are searching for clear and reliable guidance. In today's world, health information is everywhere, yet much of it is confusing, overwhelming, and sometimes misleading. My goal is to cut through that noise and present important medical topics in a way that is simple, practical, and reassuring.

Every page of this series is guided by two foundations: reliable scientific knowledge and decades of real-world clinical experience. I want you, the reader, to feel informed, confident, and empowered. Not overwhelmed. Not confused. But clear about what you can do, step by step, to improve your health.

If even one reader feels less anxious, more informed, or better prepared to take control of their health after reading these books, then this work has served its purpose.

Helping people live healthier, longer, more confident and better-informed lives remains one of the greatest privileges of my life.

Table of Contents

Introduction

Why You Should Not Ignore Acid Reflux

A Common Problem That Quietly Enters Daily Life

Acid reflux is one of those conditions that many people live with for far too long before they take it seriously. At first, it may seem small. A burning feeling after dinner. A sour taste in the mouth. A need to clear the throat. A cough that comes and goes. A restless night after a heavy meal.

Because the symptoms often begin gently, many people dismiss them. They blame the food, stress, age, a busy schedule, or one bad night of sleep. They adjust a little, ignore a little, and carry on.

That is exactly why reflux becomes such a stubborn problem. It does not always arrive dramatically. It often settles into daily life quietly, then slowly begins to control it.

When "Just Acidity" Stops Being Small

Occasional reflux can happen to almost anyone. A rich meal, eating too late, lying down too soon after dinner, or overeating at a celebration can bring on symptoms even in otherwise healthy people.

But when reflux becomes frequent, keeps returning, disturbs sleep, affects food choices, or begins to interfere with comfort and confidence, it is no longer a small problem. At that point, it deserves proper attention.

Many people continue to suffer because they keep telling themselves the same thing:

"It is nothing serious. It will settle on its own."

Sometimes it does. Very often, it does not.

Persistent reflux can reduce quality of life in ways that are easy to underestimate. It can make eating less enjoyable, nights less restful, mornings less fresh, and daily life less comfortable. Over time, it may also lead to complications that could have been prevented with earlier care.

The Good News: This Is a Condition Yo

u Can Control

Now let me share the most reassuring part.

Acid reflux is usually manageable. In many people, symptoms improve greatly with the right combination of simple lifestyle changes, better eating habits, correct use of medication, and proper medical guidance when needed.

I have seen many patients struggle with reflux for years, only to feel much better once they finally understood what was happening and started managing it in a practical, consistent way.

That is an important message to remember from the beginning of this book:

you are not powerless here.

In fact, your daily habits, your awareness, and your willingness to make a few thoughtful changes can make a remarkable difference.

Reflux Is Not Always What People Think It Is

Many people think acid reflux means one thing only: heartburn.

But reflux is often more varied than that.

Some people have the classic burning in the chest. Others feel food or fluid coming back up. Some develop a chronic cough, throat irritation, hoarseness, a bitter taste, or disturbed sleep. Some notice symptoms mainly at night. A few do not describe burning at all, yet still have significant reflux.

This is one reason why reflux is sometimes misunderstood, overlooked, or mistaken for something else.

It is also important to remember the opposite. Not every symptom in the chest, throat, or upper abdomen is caused by reflux. That is why understanding the full picture matters so much. Good treatment begins with clarity.

What Makes Reflux So Frustrating

Reflux is frustrating because it does not affect only the stomach or the esophagus. It affects daily living.

It changes how people eat.

It changes how they sleep.

It changes how they travel, exercise, socialize, and sometimes even how they speak.

Some patients grow anxious about every meal. Some become overly fearful of medication. Others try to manage the problem by avoiding more and more foods, yet still do not feel better. Many become confused because they hear too much conflicting advice.

This book has been written to clear away that confusion.

What This Book Will Help You Do

I have written this book in the same spirit in which I speak to my patients: clearly, practically, and without unnecessary medical complexity.

In the pages ahead, you will learn what acid reflux, heartburn, and GERD really mean. You will understand why reflux happens, how to recognize its different symptoms, and which warning signs should never be ignored. You will learn which lifestyle changes truly help, how medications should be used properly, what to do if symptoms are not improving, and how to reduce the risk of long-term problems.

Most importantly, this book is designed to help you move from confusion to control.

My goal is not simply to give you information. My goal is to help you use that information in real life.

A Calm, Practical, and Balanced Approach

This is not a book of fear. It is not a book of extreme restrictions. And it is not a book that asks you to live with unnecessary anxiety about every bite of food or every tablet of medicine.

Instead, this is a practical guide.

You will find realistic advice, clear explanations, and a steady step-by-step approach. You will learn how to make sensible decisions, how to recognize what matters most, and how to work with your doctor when needed.

That balanced approach is important. Most people with reflux do not have a dangerous disease. At the same time, ongoing symptoms should not be ignored. The best path lies between carelessness and fear.

Why Understanding Gives You Power

One truth has become clearer to me over the years than almost anything else in medicine: patients do best when they understand their condition.

When people understand what is happening in their bodies, they notice patterns more clearly. They ask better questions. They use treatment more effectively. They avoid myths, confusion, and unnecessary worry.

That is what I want this book to do for you.

I want it to help you understand your symptoms, regain confidence, and take sensible control of your health.

Chapter Summary

Acid reflux is common, but it should not be dismissed when it becomes frequent, persistent, or troublesome. What begins as an occasional annoyance can slowly interfere with comfort, sleep, food choices, and quality of life. The encouraging news is that reflux is usually manageable with the right understanding, practical lifestyle changes, and proper treatment.

Action Plan

For the next several days, begin paying close attention to your symptoms.

Notice:

- when they occur
- what you had eaten beforehand
- whether they are worse after lying down
- whether they disturb your sleep

Do not try to change everything at once. First, observe carefully. Awareness is the beginning of control.

Transition to Chapter 1

Now that you understand why acid reflux deserves attention, let us begin with the basics.

In the next chapter, we will clearly understand what acid reflux, heartburn, and GERD really mean, and why knowing the difference is so important.

Chapter 1

Acid Reflux, Heartburn, and GERD

Why Getting the Basics Right Matters

In my daily practice, I often notice one common problem.

Patients use the terms *acid reflux*, *heartburn*, and *GERD* as if they all mean the same thing.

They do not.

At first glance, this may seem like a small confusion. But in reality, this is where misunderstanding begins. When these terms are not clear, patients struggle to understand their condition, their symptoms, and even their treatment.

So before we go any further, let us make this simple, clear, and practical.

Acid Reflux — The Process

Acid reflux is not a disease. It is a process.

It happens when stomach contents, including acid, flow backward into the esophagus.

Normally, food travels in one direction, from the mouth to the stomach. At the lower end of the esophagus, there is a natural valve called the lower esophageal sphincter.

This valve:

- Opens to allow food into the stomach
- Closes to keep stomach contents from coming back up

When this valve becomes weak, or relaxes at the wrong time, stomach contents can move upward.

This backward flow is called acid reflux.

It can happen occasionally in anyone, especially after a heavy meal or when lying down soon after eating.

Heartburn — The Symptom

Heartburn is the most common symptom of acid reflux.

It is usually described as:

- A burning sensation in the chest
- Discomfort behind the breastbone
- A feeling that may rise toward the throat

Despite its name, heartburn has nothing to do with the heart. It is caused by irritation of the esophagus by stomach acid.

The intensity can vary. Some people feel mild discomfort. Others feel significant pain.

Heartburn often:

- Occurs after meals
- Worsens when lying down
- Is triggered by certain foods or habits

GERD — The Condition

GERD stands for gastroesophageal reflux disease.

This is not just a symptom. It is a condition.

GERD occurs when acid reflux:

- Happens frequently
- Causes troublesome symptoms
- Or leads to damage in the esophagus

In simple terms:

- Occasional reflux is common
- Frequent or persistent reflux is GERD

This distinction is important because GERD usually requires a more structured and consistent approach to treatment.

How the Body Normally Prevents Reflux

Your body has several natural defenses against reflux.

These include:

- The lower esophageal sphincter acting as a barrier
- The diaphragm supporting this valve
- The natural angle between the esophagus and stomach
- Gravity, especially when you are upright

When these systems work well, reflux is minimal.

When they become weak or disrupted, reflux becomes more likely.

Occasional Reflux Versus a Chronic Problem

Almost everyone experiences reflux at some point.

A large meal, eating late at night, or lying down too soon can trigger temporary symptoms.

This type of reflux is usually short-lived and not a cause for concern.

But when symptoms:

- Occur frequently
- Interfere with daily life
- Disturb sleep

It is no longer just occasional reflux.

At that point, it is considered GERD.

Why Reflux Differs From Person to Person

You may wonder why some people can eat almost anything without symptoms, while others struggle with even small changes.

The answer lies in individual differences.

These include:

- Strength of the lower esophageal sphincter
- Body weight and abdominal pressure
- Eating habits and meal timing
- Sensitivity of the esophagus
- Presence of conditions such as hiatal hernia

Each person has a unique combination of these factors.

That is why reflux varies so much from one individual to another.

A Simple Way to Remember

If you ever feel confused, remember this:

- **Acid reflux** is the process
- **Heartburn** is the symptom
- **GERD** is the condition

This simple understanding will guide you through the rest of the book.

Why This Clarity Helps You

When you understand these differences:

- You recognize your symptoms more accurately
- You avoid unnecessary worry
- You make better decisions about treatment
- You communicate more clearly with your doctor

This clarity is the foundation for everything that follows.

Chapter Summary

Acid reflux is the backward flow of stomach contents into the esophagus. Heartburn is the burning sensation caused by this reflux. GERD is a condition in which reflux becomes frequent, troublesome, or leads to complications.

Understanding these differences is the first and most important step toward proper diagnosis and effective treatment.

Action Plan

Take a moment to reflect:

- Do your symptoms occur occasionally or frequently?
- Do they affect your sleep or daily routine?
- Do they appear after meals or when lying down?

Write down your observations. This will help you understand your condition more clearly.

What Are Acid Reflux, Heartburn, and GERD?

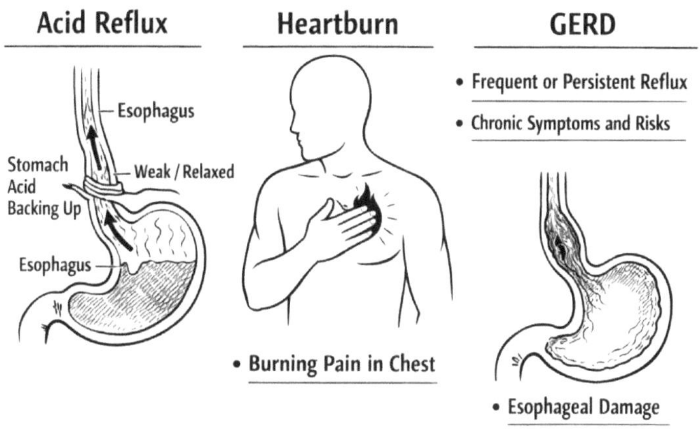

Occasional Reflux is Common – Persistent GERD Needs Attention.

Transition to Chapter 2

Now that you clearly understand what acid reflux, heartburn, and GERD mean, the next step is to understand why these problems occur. In the next chapter, we will explore the real causes of acid reflux and the factors that increase your risk.

Chapter 2

Why Acid Reflux Happens

Looking Beyond "Food" as the Only Cause

When patients come to me with reflux, the first thing they usually say is,

"Doctor, I think it is because of spicy or oily food."

Food does play a role. But in most cases, it is not the whole story.

Acid reflux develops because of a combination of factors. These include how your body functions, how you eat, your daily habits, and certain physical changes.

When you understand these causes clearly, you stop guessing and start managing your condition more effectively.

The Lower Esophageal Sphincter — The Key Valve

At the center of reflux is a small but very important structure called the lower esophageal sphincter, or LES.

Think of it as a gate between the esophagus and the stomach.

Its job is simple:

- It opens to allow food into the stomach
- It closes to keep stomach contents from coming back up

Reflux occurs when this valve:

- Becomes weak
- Relaxes at the wrong time
- Does not close completely

Even brief relaxation at the wrong time can allow acid to move upward and cause symptoms.

Hiatal Hernia — When Anatomy Changes

In some individuals, part of the stomach moves upward through the diaphragm. This is called a hiatal hernia.

When this happens:

- The support for the lower esophageal sphincter is reduced
- The valve does not function effectively
- Reflux becomes more frequent

Not everyone with reflux has a hiatal hernia. But when it is present, symptoms are often more persistent.

Excess Body Weight — A Major Contributor

Excess weight is one of the most important factors in reflux.

When weight increases:

- Pressure inside the abdomen rises
- The stomach is pushed upward
- The natural barrier becomes weaker

As a result, acid is more likely to move into the esophagus.

The encouraging part is this:

Even modest weight loss can lead to noticeable improvement.

Pregnancy — A Temporary Cause

Reflux is very common during pregnancy.

This happens due to:

- Hormonal changes that relax the LES
- Increased abdominal pressure from the growing uterus

Symptoms often become more noticeable in later stages of pregnancy.

In most cases, they improve after delivery.

Smoking — An Important but Overlooked Factor

Smoking affects reflux in several ways.

It can:

- Weaken the lower esophageal sphincter
- Reduce saliva, which helps neutralize acid
- Irritate the esophagus

For patients who smoke, quitting can significantly improve symptoms.

Eating Habits and Daily Routine

Often, the problem is not just what you eat, but how you eat.

Habits that increase reflux include:

- Eating large meals
- Eating too quickly
- Lying down soon after eating
- Eating late at night

These habits increase pressure in the stomach and make reflux more likely.

Medications That Can Worsen Reflux

Some commonly used medications can contribute to reflux.

These include:

- Certain blood pressure medications
- Sedatives
- Some asthma medications

- Pain relievers such as NSAIDs

These medications may relax the LES or irritate the esophagus.

If you are taking these medicines, do not stop them on your own. Instead, discuss with your doctor whether adjustments are needed.

Individual Sensitivity — Why Symptoms Differ

Not everyone experiences reflux in the same way.

Some people feel severe symptoms with small amounts of reflux. Others may have significant reflux but fewer symptoms.

This is due to differences in sensitivity of the esophagus.

This is also why treatment needs to be individualized.

Putting It All Together

In most patients, reflux is not caused by a single factor.

It is usually a combination of:

- Valve function
- Body weight
- Eating habits
- Lifestyle factors
- Individual sensitivity

That is why effective treatment addresses multiple areas at the same time.

A Practical Way to Think About It

Instead of asking, "What is the one cause of my reflux?" ask:

"What are the factors in my life that are contributing to it?"

This shift in thinking leads to better control.

Chapter Summary

Acid reflux occurs when the natural barrier between the stomach and esophagus does not function properly. This may be due to a weak valve, hiatal hernia, excess weight, pregnancy, smoking, certain medications, and daily habits.

Most patients have more than one contributing factor. Understanding these causes helps guide practical and effective treatment.

Action Plan

Take a few minutes to reflect:

- Do you eat late or lie down soon after meals?
- Do you have excess weight?
- Do you smoke?
- Are you taking medications that may worsen reflux?

Identify one or two factors you can begin to change this week.

Causes of Acid Reflux

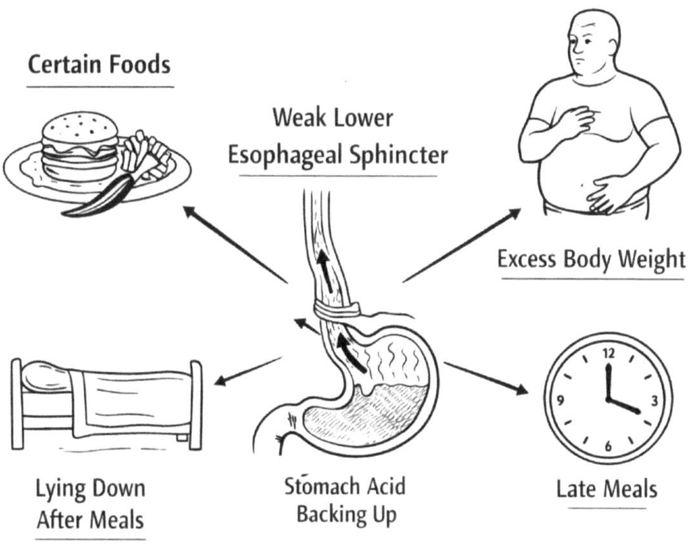

Multiple Factors Often *Contribute to* Acid Reflux.

Transition to Chapter 3

Now that you understand why acid reflux happens, the next step is to recognize how it presents in real life.

In the next chapter, we will explore the full range of symptoms, including those that are often overlooked.

Chapter 3
Recognizing the Symptoms

Why Many Patients Miss the Diagnosis

When most people think about acid reflux, they think of one symptom: heartburn.

But in real life, reflux does not always present in such a clear and familiar way.

In my practice, I have seen many patients who never complained of burning in the chest. Instead, they described a persistent cough, throat irritation, hoarseness, or a vague discomfort after meals. Some were treated repeatedly for allergies or infections before reflux was even considered.

This is why understanding the full range of symptoms is so important.

When you recognize the pattern early, you can avoid confusion, unnecessary treatment, and prolonged discomfort.

Heartburn — The Classic Symptom

Heartburn remains the most common symptom of reflux.

It is usually described as:

- A burning sensation in the chest
- Discomfort behind the breastbone
- A feeling that may rise toward the throat

It often:

- Occurs after meals
- Worsens when lying down
- Is triggered by certain foods or overeating

The intensity can vary. Some people feel mild warmth, while others experience significant discomfort.

Regurgitation — A Symptom Many Overlook

Regurgitation is another key symptom, but patients often do not recognize it as reflux.

You may notice:

- A sour or bitter taste in the mouth
- Food or fluid coming back up
- A sensation of something rising into the throat

This can be unpleasant and sometimes embarrassing, especially in social situations.

Chest Discomfort — Not Always Burning

Reflux-related chest discomfort does not always feel like burning.

Some patients describe:

- Pressure or tightness
- A dull ache after meals
- Discomfort that comes and goes

This can be confusing, especially because chest discomfort may also be related to the heart.

It is important not to assume the cause without proper evaluation.

Difficulty or Discomfort While Swallowing

Changes in swallowing should always be noted.

You may feel:

- Food moving slowly
- A sensation of food getting stuck
- Discomfort while swallowing

These symptoms may suggest irritation or narrowing of the esophagus and should be taken seriously.

Throat Symptoms — Easy to Miss

Reflux can affect the throat in subtle ways.

Patients often report:

- Frequent throat clearing
- A sensation of something stuck in the throat
- Mild irritation or scratchiness
- Hoarseness

These symptoms are often worse in the morning and are commonly mistaken for allergies or a minor infection.

Chronic Cough — An Unexpected Clue

A persistent cough without a clear cause can sometimes be related to reflux.

This type of cough:

- Is usually dry
- May worsen at night
- Does not respond well to usual treatments

Reflux may not be the only cause, but it can be an important factor.

Nighttime Symptoms — A Key Warning Pattern

Symptoms that occur at night are particularly important.

These may include:

- Burning that wakes you from sleep
- Coughing or choking during the night
- Poor or interrupted sleep

Nighttime symptoms often suggest more significant reflux and deserve attention.

Less Obvious Symptoms

Some symptoms are vague and easily overlooked.

These include:

- Bloating
- Mild upper abdominal discomfort
- Nausea

While these alone do not confirm reflux, they may be part of the overall picture.

Why Patterns Matter More Than Individual Symptoms

No single symptom tells the whole story.

What matters most is the pattern:

- When do your symptoms occur?
- What seems to trigger them?
- Do they improve with treatment?

Understanding your pattern is the key to proper diagnosis and effective management.

A Practical Perspective

Instead of focusing on one symptom, look at the overall picture.

Reflux is often recognized not by one sign, but by a combination of symptoms that follow a consistent pattern.

Chapter Summary

Acid reflux can present in many different ways. While heartburn and regurgitation are the most common symptoms, others include chest discomfort, swallowing difficulty, throat irritation, chronic cough, and nighttime symptoms.

Recognizing patterns is more important than focusing on a single symptom.

Action Plan

Take a few minutes to reflect:

- What symptoms do you experience most often?
- When do they occur?
- Are they worse after meals or at night?

Write these down. This simple step will help you understand your condition more clearly.

Transition to Chapter 4

Now that you understand how reflux can present, the next important step is to recognize which symptoms require urgent attention.

In the next chapter, we will discuss the warning signs that should never be ignored.

Chapter 4

Warning Signs You Must Never Ignore

Why This Chapter Is Crucial

So far, we have discussed symptoms that are common and often manageable.

But there is another side you must understand clearly.

Certain symptoms are warning signs. They may suggest complications of reflux or, at times, a completely different and more serious condition.

In my practice, I always give the same advice:

Stay calm, but do not delay.

Recognizing these signs early can prevent serious problems and ensure timely care.

Chest Pain — Always Treat With Caution

Chest discomfort is common in reflux. But it can also be a sign of heart disease.

This is one situation where assumptions can be dangerous.

Be especially alert if the pain:

- Feels like pressure, tightness, or heaviness
- Spreads to the arm, neck, or jaw
- Occurs with exertion
- Is associated with sweating, shortness of breath, or dizziness

If there is any doubt, treat chest pain as a possible heart problem first and seek urgent medical care.

It is always better to be cautious.

Difficulty Swallowing (Dysphagia)

If you feel that food is getting stuck while swallowing, do not ignore it.

This may suggest:

- Narrowing of the esophagus
- Ongoing inflammation
- Structural changes

This symptom usually requires further evaluation and should not be delayed.

Pain While Swallowing (Odynophagia)

Pain during swallowing is another important warning sign.

Patients may describe:

- Sharp pain when swallowing
- Burning or discomfort with each swallow

This may indicate irritation, ulcers, or infection in the esophagus.

Prompt medical attention is important.

Vomiting Blood or Black Stools

These are clear signs of possible bleeding in the digestive tract.

You may notice:

- Vomit that appears red or like coffee grounds
- Black, tarry stools

These symptoms should be treated as urgent.

Immediate medical evaluation is necessary.

Unexplained Weight Loss

Losing weight without trying should never be ignored.

It becomes more concerning when it occurs along with:

- Difficulty swallowing
- Persistent symptoms

- Loss of appetite

This is a signal that further evaluation is needed.

Persistent Vomiting or Severe Symptoms

Occasional nausea can occur with reflux.

But persistent vomiting is not typical.

Be alert if:

- You are unable to keep food down
- Symptoms are rapidly worsening
- Medications are not helping at all

These situations require prompt medical attention.

A Change in Your Usual Symptoms

Sometimes the most important clue is change.

Be cautious if:

- Symptoms become more frequent
- Discomfort becomes more intense
- New symptoms appear

Even if your symptoms were mild before, a noticeable change should not be ignored.

Putting This Into Perspective

Most cases of acid reflux are not dangerous.

But warning signs are different. They are your body's way of asking for attention.

Recognizing these signals early allows timely diagnosis and appropriate treatment.

Chapter Summary

While most reflux symptoms are manageable, certain warning signs require urgent attention. These include chest pain, difficulty or pain while swallowing, vomiting blood, black stools, unexplained weight loss, persistent vomiting, and worsening symptoms.

These signs may indicate complications or other serious conditions and should never be ignored.

Action Plan

Ask yourself:

- Do I have difficulty swallowing?
- Have I lost weight without trying?
- Have my symptoms changed recently?
- Have I experienced severe or unusual discomfort?

If the answer is yes, seek medical evaluation promptly.

Transition to Chapter 5

Now that you understand the warning signs, the next important step is to recognize that not all symptoms are caused by reflux.

In the next chapter, we will discuss conditions that can mimic GERD and why getting the correct diagnosis matters.

Chapter 5

When It Is Not GERD

Why This Chapter Matters More Than You Think

By now, you understand reflux well. But here is a truth I want you to remember:

Not every burning sensation, chest discomfort, cough, or throat symptom is due to reflux.

In my practice, I have seen many patients treated for GERD for months without real improvement. The reason was simple. The diagnosis was not correct.

When the diagnosis is not right, even the best treatment will not work.

This chapter will help you recognize situations where something else may be responsible.

Functional Heartburn — When Tests Are Normal

Some patients have symptoms that feel exactly like heartburn.

Yet when we evaluate them:

- The esophagus looks normal
- Acid exposure is not significantly increased

This condition is called **functional heartburn**.

In this situation, the issue is not excess acid. It is increased sensitivity of the esophagus.

These patients often do not respond well to standard acid-reducing medications.

Reflux Hypersensitivity — When Small Changes Feel Large

In some cases, reflux is present, but only in small amounts.

However, the esophagus is highly sensitive.

Even minimal reflux can cause noticeable symptoms.

This condition is called **reflux hypersensitivity**.

It behaves differently from typical GERD and often needs a more individualized approach.

Indigestion and Peptic Ulcer Disease

Upper abdominal discomfort is often mistaken for reflux.

Patients may describe:

- Fullness after meals
- Upper abdominal pain
- Nausea

These symptoms may be due to indigestion or ulcers rather than reflux.

Careful evaluation helps distinguish between these conditions.

Eosinophilic Esophagitis — Often Overlooked

This is an inflammatory condition of the esophagus, often related to allergies.

Patients may experience:

- Difficulty swallowing
- Food getting stuck
- Chest discomfort

It can resemble reflux but requires a completely different treatment approach.

Recognizing it early is important.

Esophageal Motility Disorders

The esophagus normally moves food downward in a coordinated way.

In some conditions, this movement is disturbed.

Patients may notice:

- Difficulty swallowing
- Chest discomfort
- A sensation that food is not moving properly

These disorders are less common but important, especially when symptoms do not improve with usual treatment.

Heart-Related Chest Pain — Never Miss This

This is one of the most critical distinctions.

Chest discomfort may be related to the heart rather than reflux.

Be especially cautious if:

- Pain occurs with exertion
- It is associated with shortness of breath
- It radiates to the arm, neck, or jaw

Never assume chest pain is due to reflux without proper evaluation.

Other Conditions That Can Mimic Reflux

Several other conditions can overlap with reflux symptoms:

- Gallbladder disease
- Pancreatic conditions

- Anxiety-related symptoms
- Throat and voice disorders

These may not be common, but they become important when symptoms do not follow a typical pattern.

Why Symptoms Alone Can Be Misleading

Many people try to diagnose themselves based on symptoms alone.

This may work in simple cases, but not always.

If symptoms:

- Do not improve with treatment
- Feel unusual
- Persist for a long time

Further evaluation is necessary.

A Practical Way to Think About It

Instead of assuming every symptom is reflux, ask:

"Does my condition behave like typical reflux?"

If the answer is not clear, it is time to look deeper.

This approach avoids unnecessary treatment and leads to better results.

Other Medical Conditions with Similar Symptoms

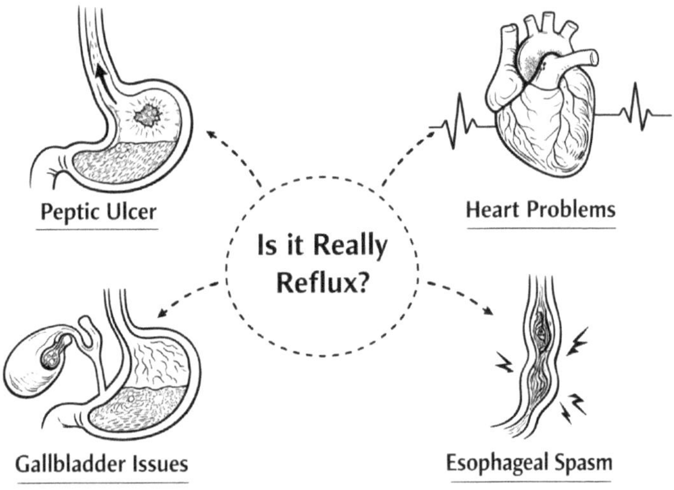

Discuss Persistent or Unusual Symptoms with Your Doctor.

Chapter Summary

Not all symptoms that resemble acid reflux are caused by GERD. Conditions such as functional heartburn, reflux hypersensitivity, ulcers, eosinophilic esophagitis, motility disorders, and heart disease can mimic reflux.

Accurate diagnosis is essential for effective treatment.

Action Plan

Reflect on your situation:

- Have your symptoms improved with reflux treatment?
- Do they follow a typical pattern?
- Have they persisted despite proper medication use?

If symptoms are not improving, discuss further evaluation with your doctor.

Transition to Chapter 6

Now that you understand that symptoms can sometimes be misleading, the next step is to see how doctors confirm the diagnosis.

In the next chapter, we will discuss the tests used to evaluate GERD and how they guide treatment decisions.

Chapter 6
How Doctors Confirm the Diagnosis

Why Diagnosis Should Not Be Based on Guesswork

Many people believe that diagnosing acid reflux is simple.

You have symptoms, you take a medicine, and if you feel better, that must be the answer.

In many cases, this approach works.

But not always.

Some patients improve only partially. Others do not improve at all. A few have symptoms that are not typical. In these situations, we need a more careful and structured approach.

A correct diagnosis is the foundation of effective treatment.

When Symptoms Alone May Be Enough

For many patients with typical symptoms such as heartburn and regurgitation, doctors may begin treatment based on symptoms alone.

This is practical and often effective.

If symptoms improve with treatment, it supports the diagnosis of GERD.

However, this approach works best when:

- Symptoms are clear and typical
- There are no warning signs
- The response to treatment is good

If any of these are not present, further evaluation may be needed.

When Testing Becomes Necessary

There are situations where symptoms alone are not enough.

Further testing is usually considered when:

- Symptoms do not improve with treatment
- Symptoms are unusual or unclear
- Warning signs are present
- Long-term treatment is being planned
- Surgery or procedures are being considered

In these cases, testing provides clarity and prevents unnecessary or incorrect treatment.

Upper Endoscopy — Looking Directly Inside

Upper endoscopy is one of the most useful tests.

A thin, flexible tube with a camera is gently passed through the mouth into the esophagus and stomach.

This allows the doctor to:

- Look for inflammation
- Detect ulcers or narrowing
- Identify complications such as Barrett's esophagus
- Rule out other conditions

The procedure is usually done with sedation and is generally safe and well tolerated.

pH Monitoring — Measuring Acid Exposure

Sometimes, we need to measure how much acid is actually reaching the esophagus.

This is done through pH monitoring.

A small device records acid levels over a period of time, usually 24 hours or longer.

This test helps:

- Confirm whether reflux is present
- Correlate symptoms with acid exposure
- Evaluate cases where the diagnosis is uncertain

Impedance Testing — Detecting More Than Acid

Not all reflux is strongly acidic.

Some patients have weakly acidic or non-acid reflux.

Impedance testing can detect:

- Movement of liquid and gas in the esophagus
- Both acid and non-acid reflux

This is especially helpful in patients who continue to have symptoms despite treatment.

Esophageal Manometry — Evaluating Function

The esophagus moves food downward through coordinated muscle contractions.

Manometry measures how well these muscles are working.

It helps assess:

- Swallowing coordination
- Strength of contractions
- Function of the lower esophageal sphincter

This test is often used before surgery or when a motility disorder is suspected.

Testing On or Off Medication — Why It Matters

One important detail is whether testing is done while you are taking medication or after stopping it.

- Testing off medication helps confirm the presence of reflux
- Testing on medication helps understand persistent symptoms

Your doctor decides this based on your situation.

How Test Results Guide Treatment

Testing is not done just to collect information.

It helps answer important questions:

- Is reflux truly present?
- Is it acid or non-acid reflux?
- Is there damage to the esophagus?
- Could another condition be responsible?

The answers guide the next steps in treatment.

A Thoughtful Approach Leads to Better Outcomes

Instead of guessing, a structured approach allows us to:

- Confirm the diagnosis
- Understand the condition clearly
- Choose the most appropriate treatment

This leads to better results and avoids unnecessary treatments.

How Diagnosis is Made

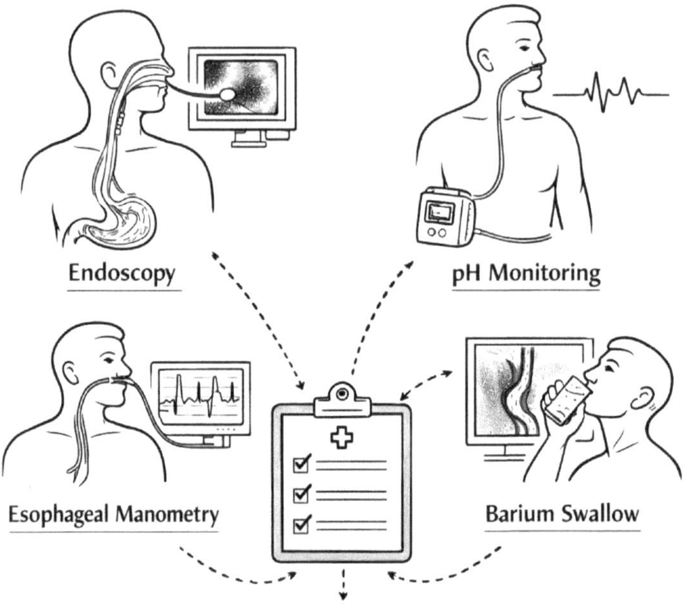

Diagnosis Depends on
Evaluation of Symptoms and Tests.

Chapter Summary

GERD can often be diagnosed based on symptoms, especially when they are typical and respond to treatment. However, when symptoms are unclear, persistent, or associated with warning signs, further testing is needed.

Tests such as endoscopy, pH monitoring, impedance testing, and manometry help confirm the diagnosis and guide treatment decisions.

Action Plan

Think about your situation:

- Have your symptoms improved with treatment?
- Are your symptoms typical or unusual?
- Have you undergone any diagnostic testing?

If your symptoms are not improving or are unclear, discuss further evaluation with your doctor.

Transition to Chapter 7

Now that you understand how GERD is diagnosed, the next step is to focus on one of the most practical areas of control: food and eating habits.

In the next chapter, we will explore how diet influences reflux and how to make simple, effective changes.

Chapter 7

Food and Eating Habits — What Truly Triggers

Moving Beyond the Fear of Food

When patients first come to me, many are already worried about food.

Some have stopped eating several things. Some avoid spices, others avoid coffee, and a few have reduced their diet so much that eating has become stressful rather than enjoyable.

This is not the right approach.

Food does play a role in reflux, but fear of food often makes the situation worse. The goal is not restriction. The goal is understanding.

The Real Issue — Pressure Inside the Stomach

The most important factor is not a single food item. It is what happens inside the stomach after you eat.

When the stomach becomes too full:

- Pressure increases
- The natural valve is stretched
- Acid is more likely to move upward

This is why large meals are one of the most common triggers of reflux.

Portion Size Matters More Than You Think

Many patients focus only on *what* they eat and ignore *how much* they eat.

Even healthy food can cause reflux if eaten in large quantities.

A practical approach is:

- Eat smaller portions
- Avoid going from very hungry to very full
- Stop eating before you feel heavy

This simple change often brings significant relief.

Meal Timing — A Key Factor

When you eat is just as important as what you eat.

Late meals are a major contributor to reflux.

If you eat and then lie down soon after:

- The stomach remains full
- Digestion is still active
- Acid can easily move upward

Allowing enough time between your last meal and sleep can make a noticeable difference.

Common Food Triggers — Not the Same for Everyone

Certain foods are more likely to trigger symptoms in some people.

These include:

- Fatty or fried foods
- Spicy foods
- Chocolate
- Coffee and tea
- Alcohol
- Carbonated drinks
- Citrus fruits
- Tomato-based foods

But here is the key point:

Not all of these affect everyone.

Personalizing Your Diet

Instead of avoiding everything, focus on your own experience.

Ask yourself:

- Which foods clearly trigger my symptoms?
- Which foods do not affect me?

A personalized approach is more practical, more effective, and easier to maintain.

How You Eat Is Just as Important

Eating habits play a major role.

Helpful practices include:

- Eating slowly
- Chewing food well
- Sitting upright while eating
- Avoiding distractions that lead to overeating

These simple habits reduce pressure in the stomach and improve digestion.

The Role of Beverages

What you drink also matters.

Some beverages may worsen symptoms, especially when taken in large amounts.

Be mindful of:

- Caffeinated drinks
- Alcohol
- Carbonated beverages

Moderation and observation are more useful than complete avoidance.

Avoiding Over-Restriction

One of the biggest mistakes I see is over-restriction.

Patients avoid too many foods, yet symptoms continue.

This leads to frustration and reduced quality of life.

A balanced approach works better:

- Identify triggers
- Modify intake
- Maintain a varied and enjoyable diet

Using a Food and Symptom Diary

A simple and powerful tool is a food diary.

For one to two weeks, note:

- What you eat
- When you eat
- When symptoms occur

Patterns often become clear when written down.

This helps you make targeted changes instead of guessing.

A Practical Way Forward

Instead of asking, “What should I stop eating?” ask:

“What changes in my eating pattern will help me feel better?”

This shift makes management realistic and sustainable.

Chapter Summary

Food plays an important role in reflux, but portion size, meal timing, and eating habits are equally important. Large meals and late-night eating are common triggers.

A personalized and balanced approach works better than strict and unnecessary restrictions.

Action Plan

For the next two weeks:

- Eat smaller portions
- Avoid eating within 2–3 hours of bedtime
- Keep a simple food and symptom diary
- Identify one or two personal triggers

Focus on consistency, not perfection.

Transition to Chapter 8

Food is only one part of the picture.

In the next chapter, we will explore lifestyle changes such as weight, sleep, posture, and daily habits that can make a powerful difference in controlling reflux.

Chapter 8

Lifestyle Changes That Truly Work

Why Daily Habits Make the Biggest Difference

When people think about treating acid reflux, they often think first about medicines.

But over many years in practice, I have seen something very clear.

Patients who do well in the long run are not always the ones on the strongest medication. They are the ones who make steady, practical changes in their daily habits.

These changes are simple. They do not require special equipment or complicated plans. But when followed consistently, they can make a powerful difference.

Weight — One of the Most Important Factors

Excess body weight is a major contributor to reflux.

When weight increases:

- Pressure inside the abdomen rises
- The stomach is pushed upward
- The natural valve becomes less effective

As a result, acid can move upward more easily.

The encouraging part is this:

Even modest weight loss can significantly reduce symptoms.

You do not need rapid or extreme changes. A gradual and steady approach works best.

Do Not Lie Down After Meals

This is one of the simplest and most effective habits you can adopt.

If you lie down soon after eating:

- The stomach is still full
- Digestion is ongoing
- Acid can easily move upward

Try to stay upright for at least 2 to 3 hours after meals.

Even a gentle walk after eating can help.

Sleep Position — Let Gravity Work for You

Nighttime reflux is often worse because gravity is no longer helping you.

When you lie flat:

- Acid can move upward more easily
- Symptoms may become more noticeable

Elevating the head of your bed can make a meaningful difference.

Using a wedge pillow or raising the head of the bed is more effective than stacking regular pillows.

Smoking — A Strong but Modifiable Factor

Smoking affects reflux in several ways.

It can:

- Weaken the lower esophageal sphincter
- Reduce saliva, which helps neutralize acid
- Irritate the lining of the esophagus

Stopping smoking is one of the most beneficial steps you can take, not only for reflux but for your overall health.

Alcohol — Use With Awareness

Alcohol can worsen reflux in some people.

It may:

- Relax the lower esophageal sphincter
- Increase exposure of the esophagus to acid

You do not always need to eliminate alcohol completely, but

moderation and observation are important.

Posture and Daily Movements

Small physical habits during the day can influence reflux.

Helpful adjustments include:

- Avoiding tight clothing around the abdomen
- Being cautious with bending forward after meals
- Sitting upright while eating

These small changes reduce pressure on the stomach and help prevent reflux.

Building a Routine That Lasts

One common mistake is trying to change everything at once.

This often leads to frustration and inconsistency.

A better approach is:

- Start with one or two changes
- Practice them regularly
- Gradually add more as they become habits

Consistency matters more than intensity.

Why Small Changes Work

Patients often expect quick results.

But long-term improvement comes from steady habits.

Over time, these changes:

- Reduce frequency of symptoms
- Improve sleep
- Increase comfort during daily activities

This is how lasting control is achieved.

A Practical Perspective

Instead of asking, "What major change do I need?" ask:

"What small change can I start today and continue tomorrow?"

That is how real progress begins.

Chapter Summary

Lifestyle changes are a central part of managing acid reflux. Weight control, avoiding lying down after meals, improving sleep position, reducing smoking and alcohol, and maintaining good daily habits can significantly reduce symptoms.

These changes are simple but highly effective when practiced consistently.

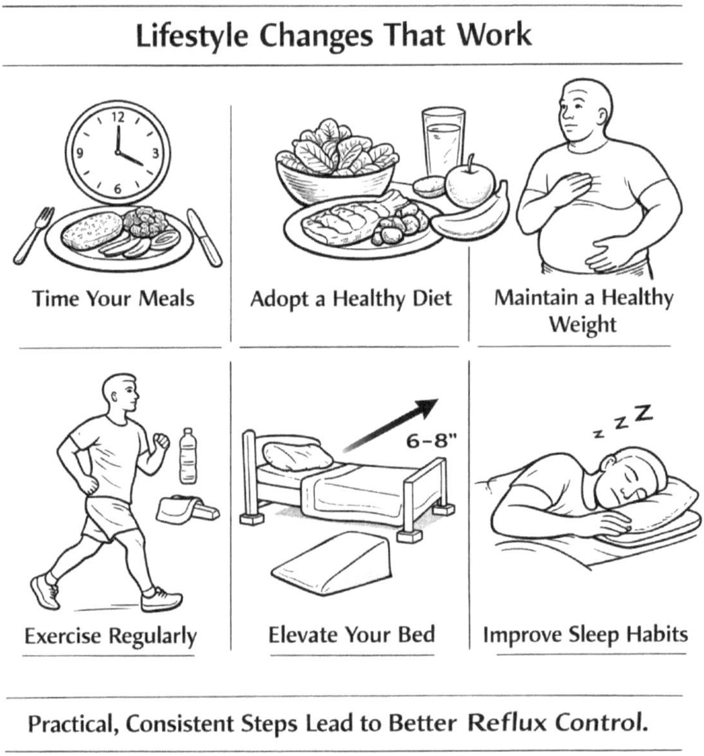
Lifestyle Changes That Work
12
3
6
9
Time Your Meals
Adopt a Healthy Diet
Maintain a Healthy Weight
6-8"
Exercise Regularly
Elevate Your Bed
Improve Sleep Habits
Practical, Consistent Steps Lead to Better Reflux Control.

Action Plan

Choose two changes to begin this week:

- Avoid lying down after meals
- Elevate the head of your bed
- Begin gradual weight reduction
- Reduce smoking or alcohol

Start small, stay consistent, and observe the difference.

Transition to Chapter 9

Even with good lifestyle habits, many patients continue to experience symptoms at night.

In the next chapter, we will focus specifically on nighttime reflux and how to manage it effectively.

Chapter 9

Nighttime Reflux — Why Symptoms Worsen at Night

Why Nights Often Become Difficult

Many patients tell me something very similar:

"Doctor, I feel okay during the day, but nights are the worst."

This is not a coincidence.

During the day, when you are upright, gravity helps keep stomach contents where they belong. At night, when you lie flat, that natural protection is reduced.

If the stomach is still full or the valve is weak, acid can move upward more easily.

That is why nighttime reflux often feels stronger, more uncomfortable, and more disruptive.

How Nighttime Reflux Affects Your Life

Nighttime reflux is not just a minor inconvenience.

It can:

- Wake you from sleep
- Cause coughing or choking
- Create a sour taste in the mouth
- Lead to poor-quality sleep

Over time, this can result in:

- Daytime fatigue
- Reduced concentration
- Irritability

Sleep and reflux are closely connected. When one is disturbed, the other suffers.

Symptoms That May Be Missed

Nighttime reflux does not always appear as classic heartburn.

You may notice:

- Frequent waking without clear reason
- Morning throat irritation
- Hoarseness on waking
- A persistent cough at night

Because these symptoms are subtle, many people do not relate them to reflux.

Late Meals — The Most Common Cause

One of the most important triggers is eating too close to bedtime.

When you go to bed with a full stomach:

- Digestion is still active
- Acid production continues
- Reflux becomes more likely

Even a healthy meal can cause symptoms if the timing is not right.

Heavy Evening Meals — A Common Mistake

Even when dinner is taken early, large or heavy meals can still cause problems.

A heavy meal:

- Stays longer in the stomach
- Increases pressure
- Promotes reflux

Keeping dinner lighter than lunch is a practical and effective strategy.

Elevating the Head of the Bed — A Simple but Powerful Step

This is one of the most effective measures for nighttime reflux.

When your upper body is elevated:

- Gravity helps keep acid down
- Reflux episodes are reduced

Use:

- Bed risers under the head of the bed
- A wedge pillow

Regular pillows are usually not sufficient because they do not maintain proper elevation of the upper body.

Your Evening Routine Matters

Small changes in your evening routine can make a big difference:

- Finish dinner at least 2–3 hours before sleep
- Avoid bending forward after meals
- Keep your routine calm and consistent

These habits improve both digestion and sleep.

When Nighttime Symptoms Need Attention

Occasional nighttime symptoms can occur.

But you should seek evaluation if:

- Symptoms occur frequently
- Sleep is regularly disturbed
- There is choking or severe discomfort

Persistent nighttime reflux often requires adjustment in treatment.

Breaking the Sleep-Reflux Cycle

Nighttime reflux can create a cycle:

Poor sleep '! increased sensitivity '! worse symptoms '! poorer sleep

Breaking this cycle is important.

Improving your sleep habits can reduce reflux, and controlling reflux can improve your sleep.

A Practical Way to Think About It

Ask yourself:

"What can I change in my evening routine that will help me sleep better?"

This simple question often leads to meaningful improvements.

Chapter Summary

Nighttime reflux occurs because lying down reduces the effect of gravity, allowing acid to move upward more easily. Late meals, heavy dinners, and poor sleep habits are common triggers.

Simple changes in meal timing, portion size, and sleep position can significantly reduce symptoms.

Action Plan

Start with these steps:

- Finish dinner at least 2–3 hours before bedtime
- Keep dinner light
- Elevate the head of your bed
- Observe your sleep quality

Small changes at night can lead to big improvements.

Transition to Chapter 10

Lifestyle changes are essential, but many patients also need medications for better control.

In the next chapter, we will discuss the different types of medicines used for reflux and how to use them effectively.

Chapter 10

Medicines That Help — Choosing Wisely and Using Them Correctly

Why Medicines Are Sometimes Necessary

By now, you have seen how much lifestyle and dietary changes can help.

But in real life, many patients still need medication, at least for a period of time.

This is not a failure. It simply means your body needs additional support.

The key point is this:

Medicines work well, but only when they are used correctly.

In my practice, I often see patients who say, "Doctor, the medicine is not helping." When we look closely, the issue is not the medicine itself, but how it is being used.

The Main Types of Medicines

There are three main groups of medicines used in acid reflux.

Understanding them will help you use them more effectively.

Antacids — Quick but Short Relief

Antacids act quickly.

They work by neutralizing stomach acid already present.

They are useful for:

- Occasional symptoms
- Mild discomfort after meals

However:

- Their effect is short
- They do not prevent reflux
- They do not heal the esophagus

Think of them as a temporary solution, not a long-term strategy.

H2 Blockers — Moderate and Useful

H2 blockers reduce the amount of acid the stomach produces.

They are helpful for:

- Mild to moderate symptoms
- Occasional nighttime symptoms

They last longer than antacids but are less powerful than PPIs.

For some patients, they are enough. For others, stronger treatment is needed.

Proton Pump Inhibitors (PPIs) — The Most Effective Option

PPIs are the most effective medications for acid reflux.

They work by significantly reducing acid production.

They are especially useful for:

- Frequent symptoms
- More severe reflux
- Inflammation of the esophagus

When used correctly, they provide consistent relief and allow healing.

Timing — The Most Important Detail

This is where many patients make mistakes.

PPIs must be taken at the right time to work properly.

For best results:

- Take them **30 to 60 minutes before breakfast**
- If prescribed twice daily, take the second dose before dinner

Taking them after meals reduces their effectiveness.

This small detail often makes a big difference.

Over-the-Counter Use — When to Be Careful

Many reflux medications are available without a prescription.

This can be helpful for short-term relief.

But problems arise when:

- Symptoms persist and are not evaluated
- Medicines are used incorrectly
- Treatment continues without a clear diagnosis

If symptoms continue, it is important to seek proper medical advice.

Side Effects — Keeping Things in Perspective

Most reflux medications are well tolerated.

Some patients may experience:

- Mild headache
- Stomach discomfort
- Changes in bowel habits

Serious side effects are uncommon.

Understanding this helps reduce unnecessary fear.

Common Mistakes That Reduce Benefit

Many patients do not get full benefit because of simple errors:

- Taking medication irregularly

- Stopping too early
- Taking PPIs at the wrong time
- Frequently switching medicines without guidance

Correcting these often improves symptoms without changing the medicine.

Medicines Are Part of a Larger Plan

Medicines are helpful, but they are not a complete solution by themselves.

They work best when combined with:

- Proper eating habits
- Lifestyle changes
- A structured treatment plan

The goal is:

- Relief of symptoms
- Healing when needed
- Long-term control with minimal medication

A Practical Way to Think About It

Instead of asking, "Which is the strongest medicine?" ask:

"How can I use the right medicine in the right way?"

That is what leads to better results.

Medications for Acid Reflux and GERD

Antacids

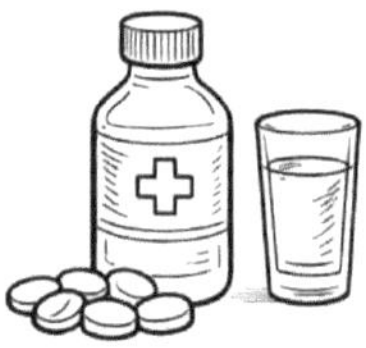

- Neutralize Stomach Acid
- Fast and Short-Acting

H2 Blockers

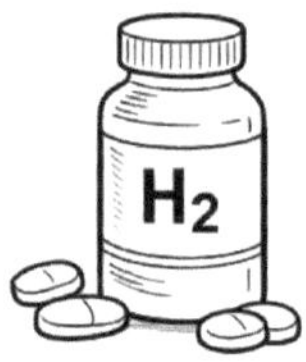

- Reduce Acid Production
- Work for Hours

Proton Pump Inhibitors

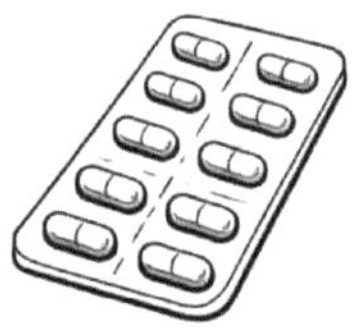

- Strongly Suppress Acid
- Most Potent and Long-Lasting

Follow Your Doctor's Instructions for Best Results.

Chapter Summary

Medications are an important part of reflux management. Antacids provide quick relief, H2 blockers reduce acid moderately, and PPIs are the most effective for frequent or severe symptoms.

Correct timing, proper use, and avoiding common mistakes are essential for success.

Action Plan

Review your current treatment:

- Are you taking your medication at the correct time?
- Are you taking it regularly?
- Have you seen improvement?

If not, focus on correct use before changing medications.

Transition to Chapter 11

Since PPIs are such an important part of treatment, they deserve a closer and more balanced discussion.

In the next chapter, we will understand their benefits, possible risks, and how to use them wisely.

Chapter 11

Proton Pump Inhibitors (PPIs) — Benefits & Risks

Why There Is So Much Confusion About PPIs

If you speak to different people about PPIs, you will hear very different opinions.

Some will tell you these medicines changed their life. Others will warn you about long-term side effects and advise you to avoid them completely.

This creates confusion and, in many cases, unnecessary fear.

Let us bring clarity.

PPIs are among the most effective medications we have for acid reflux. Like all medicines, they should be used thoughtfully. But when used correctly, they are both helpful and safe for most patients.

What Exactly Are PPIs?

PPIs, or proton pump inhibitors, reduce acid production in the stomach.

They work at the final step of acid secretion, which makes them more powerful than other acid-reducing medications.

By lowering acid levels, they:

- Reduce irritation of the esophagus
- Relieve symptoms such as heartburn and regurgitation
- Allow healing of inflammation

This is why they are often the main treatment for GERD.

What PPIs Do Well

When used properly, PPIs can provide significant benefits.

They can:

- Relieve frequent heartburn
- Improve nighttime symptoms
- Help heal inflammation of the esophagus
- Improve overall quality of life

Many patients who struggled for a long time experience clear improvement once they start using PPIs correctly.

Understanding the Concerns

Over time, concerns about PPIs have increased.

Patients often ask:

- Are these medicines safe for long-term use?
- Will they harm my body?
- Should I stop them as soon as possible?

It is important to understand that many of these concerns come from studies showing associations, not direct cause-and-effect relationships.

This means the risks are often smaller than they appear.

What We Know About Safety

For most patients, PPIs are safe when used appropriately.

Some possible concerns discussed in medical literature include:

- Reduced absorption of certain nutrients with long-term use
- Slightly increased risk of certain infections
- Possible effects on bone health in some individuals

These risks are generally small and depend on factors such as age, overall health, and duration of use.

The key is balanced use, not avoidance.

When Long-Term Use Is Appropriate

Not everyone needs long-term treatment.

However, long-term use may be appropriate in patients with:

- Frequent or severe symptoms

- Documented inflammation of the esophagus
- Barrett's esophagus

In such cases, the benefits of continued treatment usually outweigh the risks.

Using the Lowest Effective Dose

A very practical principle in medicine is:

Use the lowest dose that keeps your symptoms under control.

Many patients:

- Start with a higher dose
- Improve over time
- Gradually reduce the dose

This approach maintains benefit while minimizing unnecessary medication use.

Avoiding Sudden Stopping

One common mistake is stopping PPIs suddenly.

This can lead to:

- Temporary increase in acid production
- Return of symptoms
- Confusion and concern

Gradual reduction is usually a better approach.

Avoiding Fear-Based Decisions

Many patients stop PPIs after reading something online.

This is not the best way to make decisions.

Treatment should be based on:

- Your symptoms
- Your diagnosis
- Your response to therapy

Decisions should be thoughtful and guided, not driven by fear.

A Balanced Perspective

PPIs are not harmful when used appropriately. They are not necessary for everyone, and they are not meant to be used blindly.

They are tools.

When used correctly:

- They provide relief
- They promote healing
- They improve daily comfort

A Practical Way to Think About It

Instead of asking, "Are PPIs good or bad?" ask:

"When do I need them, and how should I use them properly?"

This approach leads to better outcomes.

Chapter Summary

PPIs are the most effective medications for acid reflux and GERD. They reduce acid production, relieve symptoms, and allow healing of the esophagus.

While concerns about long-term use exist, most risks are small. Proper use and a balanced approach are essential.

Action Plan

Review your use of PPIs:

- Are you taking them at the correct time?
- Are you using the lowest effective dose?
- Have you discussed long-term use with your doctor?

Plan to review your treatment and adjust it thoughtfully if needed.

Transition to Chapter 12

Now that you understand PPIs clearly, the next step is to learn how to adjust your treatment over time.

In the next chapter, we will discuss how to find the right treatment plan and maintain long-term control.

Chapter 12

Finding the Right Treatment Plan

Why There Is No One-Size-Fits-All Treatment

One of the most important lessons in managing acid reflux is this:

There is no single treatment plan that works for everyone.

Some patients improve with simple lifestyle changes. Others need medication for a period of time. A few may require longer-term treatment.

Your plan should be based on:

- Your symptoms
- Their frequency and severity
- Your response to treatment
- Your overall health

The goal is not just relief. The goal is a balanced, practical, and sustainable plan.

The Step-Up Approach — Starting Simple

For patients with mild or occasional symptoms, treatment often begins with simple steps.

This may include:

- Lifestyle changes
- Occasional use of antacids
- Short-term use of H2 blockers

If symptoms are controlled at this level, stronger treatment may not be necessary.

This approach avoids unnecessary medication and keeps treatment simple.

When to Move to Stronger Treatment

If symptoms become:

- Frequent
- More intense
- Disruptive to sleep or daily activities

Then stronger treatment is needed.

This usually means:

- Starting a proton pump inhibitor
- Using medication regularly rather than occasionally

The goal is to bring symptoms under control and allow healing.

The Step-Down Approach — Reducing Treatment Safely

Once symptoms improve, many patients wish to reduce or stop medication.

In many cases, this is possible.

A step-down approach may include:

- Reducing the dose
- Taking medication less frequently
- Switching to a milder option

The key is to maintain control while using the least amount of medication necessary.

Understanding Rebound Symptoms

Some patients notice a temporary increase in symptoms when stopping medication, especially PPIs.

This is called rebound acid production.

It can feel like the condition is worsening, but it is usually temporary.

Gradual reduction of medication helps prevent this problem.

Long-Term Maintenance — Finding Stability

For some patients, reflux is a long-term condition.

In such cases, the focus shifts to maintenance.

This may include:

- Continued lifestyle measures
- Low-dose or intermittent medication
- Periodic reassessment

The goal is steady control, not repeated cycles of worsening and treatment.

Avoiding Common Treatment Mistakes

Many patients struggle because of simple errors:

- Starting treatment too late
- Stopping medication too early
- Taking medication irregularly
- Changing treatment without proper guidance

A structured plan helps avoid these problems.

Working With Your Doctor

Treatment decisions are best made together with your doctor.

Important factors include:

- Your symptom pattern
- Your response to treatment
- Presence of complications
- Other medical conditions

A thoughtful, individualized approach leads to better outcomes.

Finding Your Personal Balance

Managing reflux is not about following rigid rules.

It is about finding what works for you.

The right plan is:

- Effective
- Practical
- Easy to maintain

When your plan fits your lifestyle, long-term success becomes much easier.

A Practical Way to Think About It

Instead of asking, "What is the strongest treatment?" ask:

"What is the simplest treatment that keeps my symptoms under control?"

That is the key to sustainable management.

Chapter Summary

Treatment of acid reflux should be individualized. Mild symptoms can often be managed with lifestyle changes and simple medications. More frequent symptoms require stronger treatment.

Once symptoms improve, a step-down approach helps reduce medication while maintaining control.

Action Plan

Think about your current treatment:

- Are your symptoms well controlled?
- Are you using more medication than necessary?
- Could your treatment be adjusted?

Discuss your plan with your doctor and make thoughtful changes if needed.

Transition to Chapter 13

Even with the right treatment plan, some patients continue to have symptoms.

In the next chapter, we will discuss what to do when treatment does not seem to work and how to approach this situation step by step.

Chapter 13

When Treatment Does Not Work

When Progress Feels Disappointing

Most patients improve once treatment is started correctly.

But some do not.

If you are in that situation, it can be frustrating. You may feel that nothing is working, or you may begin to worry that something more serious is going on.

Let me reassure you.

When treatment does not work, there is usually a reason. And when we identify that reason, we can correct the course.

The key is to approach the problem calmly and systematically.

Step 1: Check How You Are Taking Your Medication

This is the most common reason for poor response.

Many patients:

- Take medication at the wrong time
- Miss doses
- Stop treatment too early

For example, PPIs work best when taken before meals. If taken after eating, their effect is reduced.

Before changing medications, always check whether you are using them correctly.

Step 2: Revisit Your Daily Habits

Even the best medication cannot fully overcome poor habits.

Symptoms may persist if:

- You eat late at night
- Meals are large or irregular
- You lie down soon after eating
- Weight remains high

Treatment works best when medication and lifestyle changes go together.

Step 3: Ask an Important Question — Is This Really GERD?

If symptoms do not improve, it is important to reconsider the diagnosis.

Not all symptoms are caused by reflux.

As discussed earlier, conditions such as functional heartburn, reflux hypersensitivity, or other gastrointestinal and non-gastrointestinal problems can mimic GERD.

If symptoms:

- Do not respond to treatment
- Feel unusual
- Do not follow a clear pattern

Then the diagnosis may need to be reviewed.

Step 4: Consider Non-Acid Reflux

Not all reflux is acidic.

Some patients have reflux that is weakly acidic or non-acidic.

These patients may:

- Continue to have symptoms
- Not respond well to acid-reducing medications

Specialized testing can help identify this.

Step 5: Think About Sensitivity

In some patients, the esophagus becomes more sensitive.

Even small amounts of reflux can cause significant discomfort.

This is seen in:

- Functional heartburn
- Reflux hypersensitivity

In these situations, treatment may need to be adjusted in a different way.

Step 6: When Testing Becomes Necessary

If symptoms persist despite proper treatment, further evaluation is often needed.

Testing helps answer key questions:

- Is reflux truly present?
- What type of reflux is it?
- Is another condition responsible?

This step prevents unnecessary changes and confusion.

Step 7: Adjust Treatment Thoughtfully

Once the cause is clearer, treatment can be adjusted.

This may involve:

- Correcting medication use

- Strengthening lifestyle measures
- Changing the treatment approach
- Considering further evaluation

The goal is targeted treatment, not repeated trial and error.

Avoiding a Common Trap

Many patients, when frustrated, begin changing medications frequently or trying multiple remedies at once.

This often leads to more confusion.

A step-by-step approach is far more effective.

Staying Calm and Focused

Persistent symptoms can be discouraging, but they are not uncommon.

The important thing is not to lose direction.

With a clear and structured approach, most patients eventually find the right solution.

A Practical Way to Think About It

Instead of asking, "Why is nothing working?" ask:

"What step have I missed?"

This question often leads to the answer.

Chapter Summary

When treatment does not work, the cause is often incorrect medication use, unaddressed lifestyle factors, an incorrect diagnosis, non-acid reflux, or increased sensitivity of the esophagus.

A structured, step-by-step approach helps identify the cause and improve outcomes.

Action Plan

If your symptoms are not improving:

- Check how you are taking your medication
- Review your daily habits
- Consider whether your symptoms are typical
- Discuss further evaluation with your doctor

Focus on clarity before making changes.

Transition to Chapter 14

Reflux is not only a physical condition. The way your body and mind interact also plays an important role.

In the next chapter, we will explore how stress and anxiety influence reflux and how addressing them can improve your symptoms.

Chapter 14

Stress, Anxiety, and the Gut–Brain Connection

Looking Beyond the Physical Problem

When I ask patients about stress while discussing reflux, many are surprised.

Some even ask,

"Doctor, are you saying this is all in my mind?"

Let me make this very clear.

Your symptoms are real. Acid reflux is a physical condition.

But the way your mind and body interact can strongly influence how those symptoms are felt.

Understanding this connection can make a meaningful difference in how you experience and manage reflux.

The Gut–Brain Connection — A Simple Explanation

Your digestive system and your brain are closely linked.

They communicate constantly.

This is why:

- Stress can affect digestion
- Emotions can influence physical symptoms
- Minor discomfort can feel more intense during stressful periods

This connection is natural and well recognized.

How Stress Affects Reflux Symptoms

Stress does not always increase acid production significantly.

But it changes something equally important. It increases sensitivity.

When you are stressed:

- You become more aware of bodily sensations
- Discomfort feels stronger
- Small symptoms feel more troubling

Even mild reflux can feel quite severe during stressful times.

The Stress–Symptom Cycle

Many patients unknowingly fall into a cycle:

- Symptoms begin
- Concern and worry increase
- Stress levels rise
- Symptoms feel worse
- Anxiety grows further

This cycle can continue, making symptoms persistent and more difficult to manage.

Breaking this cycle is an important part of treatment.

Heightened Sensitivity — A Real Condition

Some individuals have increased sensitivity in the esophagus.

In these cases:

- Even small amounts of reflux cause noticeable discomfort
- Symptoms feel out of proportion to the actual reflux

This is not imaginary. It is a real and recognized condition.

Understanding this helps reduce frustration and guides appropriate treatment.

Sleep, Stress, and Reflux — A Connected Trio

Stress often affects sleep.

Poor sleep then:

- Increases sensitivity to symptoms

- Makes reflux feel worse
- Reduces your ability to cope

This creates another cycle:

Poor sleep ’! worse symptoms ’! more stress ’! poorer sleep

Improving sleep is an important part of breaking this pattern.

Simple Ways to Reduce the Impact of Stress

You do not need complicated techniques.

Start with simple steps:

- Take short breaks during the day
- Practice slow, deep breathing
- Maintain a regular sleep routine
- Engage in light physical activity
- Spend time doing something you enjoy

These small steps can help reduce the intensity of symptoms.

When Additional Support Is Needed

If stress or anxiety feels overwhelming, it should be addressed directly.

This may include:

- Speaking with a healthcare professional

- Learning structured relaxation techniques
- Seeking additional support when needed

Taking care of mental well-being is an important part of overall health.

Keeping the Right Perspective

It is important to maintain balance.

Reflux is not caused solely by stress.

But stress can make symptoms feel worse.

When both physical and emotional factors are addressed together, results are often better.

A Practical Way to Think About It

Instead of asking, "Is this stress or reflux?" ask:

"How can I reduce both the physical and emotional triggers of my symptoms?"

This approach leads to better control.

Chapter Summary

Stress and anxiety do not directly cause acid reflux, but they increase sensitivity and make symptoms feel worse. The connection between the gut and brain plays an important role in how symptoms are experienced.

The Gut-Brain Connection

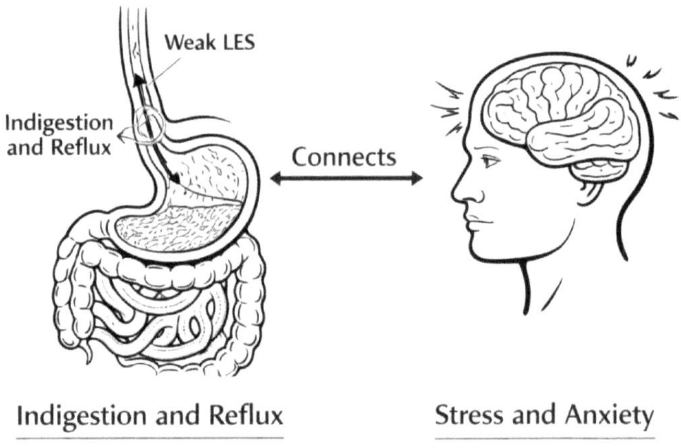

Mind and Digestive Health Are Closely Linked

Managing stress and improving sleep can significantly improve overall symptom control.

Action Plan

Take one small step this week:

- Practice deep breathing for a few minutes daily
- Improve your sleep routine
- Take a short walk regularly

Observe how your symptoms feel when your stress level is lower.

Transition to Chapter 15

Now that you understand how stress influences reflux, it is important to look at the long-term effects of uncontrolled symptoms.

In the next chapter, we will discuss what can happen if GERD is ignored over time and why proper management matters.

Chapter 15

What Happens If GERD Is Ignored

Why This Chapter Is Important

Up to this point, you have learned that acid reflux is common and, in most cases, manageable.

But there is another side that deserves clear understanding.

When reflux becomes frequent and continues for a long time without proper control, it can begin to affect the esophagus in more serious ways.

I want to emphasize something from the start.

This chapter is not meant to create fear. It is meant to give you awareness, so you can take timely and sensible action.

Inflammation of the Esophagus (Esophagitis)

The lining of the esophagus is not designed to handle repeated exposure to stomach acid.

When reflux occurs frequently:

- The lining becomes irritated
- Inflammation develops
- Symptoms may become more persistent

Patients may notice:

- More frequent heartburn
- Increased discomfort
- Pain during swallowing

If left untreated, this irritation can worsen over time.

Ulcers and Bleeding

Ongoing irritation can sometimes lead to small sores in the lining of the esophagus. These are called ulcers.

Ulcers may:

- Cause pain
- Lead to bleeding

Sometimes the bleeding is not obvious. At other times, it may appear as:

- Vomiting blood

- Dark, black stools

These signs require immediate medical attention.

Narrowing of the Esophagus (Stricture)

Repeated inflammation can lead to healing with scar formation.

Over time, this scarring may cause narrowing of the esophagus. This is called a stricture.

Patients may experience:

- Difficulty swallowing
- A feeling that food is getting stuck
- The need to eat slowly or drink liquids with meals

This can significantly affect daily eating and comfort.

Increased Sensitivity Over Time

Even without major complications, long-standing reflux can lead to increased sensitivity.

This means:

- Symptoms may occur more easily
- Discomfort may feel more intense
- Episodes may become more frequent

The longer reflux continues without control, the harder it can become to manage.

Barrett's Esophagus — A Long-Term Change

In some patients, repeated acid exposure leads to a change in the lining of the lower esophagus.

This condition is called Barrett's esophagus.

It does not develop in everyone, but when it does, it requires monitoring and follow-up.

We will discuss this in more detail in the next chapter.

Understanding Cancer Risk — With Balance

This is often the most concerning topic for patients.

Let me explain it clearly.

Most people with reflux do not develop cancer.

Barrett's esophagus can increase the risk over time, but even then, the overall risk for an individual patient remains low.

The key is awareness and appropriate follow-up, not fear.

Why Early Control Makes a Difference

The longer reflux remains uncontrolled:

- The greater the chance of complications
- The more persistent symptoms may become

On the other hand:

- Early treatment reduces inflammation

- Proper management prevents progression
- Regular follow-up ensures safety

Taking action early is always beneficial.

A Calm and Practical Perspective

It is natural to feel concerned when reading about complications.

But it is important to keep things in perspective:

- Most patients do not develop serious problems
- Effective treatments are available
- Complications develop gradually, not suddenly

Your goal is simple: recognize symptoms early and manage them properly.

A Practical Way to Think About It

Instead of asking, "What is the worst that can happen?" ask:

"What can I do now to prevent problems later?"

That is the mindset that leads to better health.

Chapter Summary

Untreated GERD can lead to complications such as inflammation, ulcers, bleeding, narrowing of the esophagus, and Barrett's esophagus. While serious complications are not common,

What Happens if GERD Is Ignored?

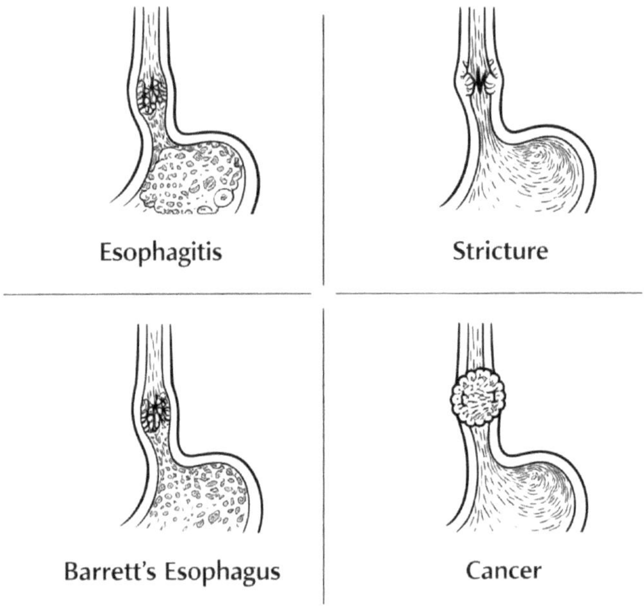

Untreated GERD Can Lead to Serious Health Problems

persistent symptoms should not be ignored.

Early and proper management helps protect long-term health.

Action Plan

Reflect on your symptoms:

- Have they been present for a long time?
- Have they gradually worsened?
- Have you been evaluated for complications?

If needed, plan a medical review to ensure proper care.

Transition to Chapter 16

Among the possible long-term effects of reflux, one condition often causes the most concern.

In the next chapter, we will discuss Barrett's esophagus in a clear and reassuring way.

Chapter 16

Barrett's Esophagus

Why This Condition Creates Concern

When patients hear the term *Barrett's esophagus*, they often become anxious.

Many immediately think of cancer. Others feel uncertain because the term sounds serious and unfamiliar.

Let me reassure you right at the beginning.

Most people with acid reflux do not develop Barrett's esophagus. And among those who do, the majority do well with proper monitoring and care.

This chapter is meant to replace fear with understanding.

What Exactly Is Barrett's Esophagus?

Barrett's esophagus is a change in the lining of the lower part of the esophagus.

Normally, the esophagus is lined with cells suited for carrying food. When this lining is exposed to acid repeatedly over a long period, the body adapts.

It replaces the normal lining with a different type that is more resistant to acid.

This protective change is called Barrett's esophagus.

Why Does This Change Occur?

This is the body's way of protecting itself from repeated irritation.

However, while the new lining is more resistant to acid, it is not the same as the original tissue.

That is why it requires monitoring over time.

Who Is More Likely to Develop It?

Barrett's esophagus does not occur in everyone with reflux.

The risk is higher in people who:

- Have long-standing reflux symptoms
- Are overweight or obese
- Are over the age of 50
- Are male
- Have a history of smoking

These are risk factors, not guarantees.

How Is It Diagnosed?

Barrett's esophagus cannot be diagnosed based on symptoms alone.

It is usually detected during an upper endoscopy.

During the procedure:

- The doctor examines the lining of the esophagus
- Small tissue samples are taken
- These samples are examined under a microscope

This confirms the diagnosis.

Understanding Dysplasia — Keeping It Simple

Sometimes, the cells in Barrett's esophagus show early changes.

These changes are called dysplasia.

They are classified as:

- No dysplasia
- Low-grade dysplasia
- High-grade dysplasia

You can think of this as a spectrum, ranging from minimal change to more advanced change.

Most patients do not have significant dysplasia.

What About Cancer Risk?

This is the most common concern.

Barrett's esophagus is associated with an increased risk of a certain type of esophageal cancer.

But it is important to understand this clearly:

The overall risk for an individual patient is low.

Most people with Barrett's esophagus never develop cancer.

The purpose of diagnosis and monitoring is early detection, not alarm.

Why Regular Follow-Up Is Important

If Barrett's esophagus is diagnosed, your doctor may recommend periodic endoscopy.

This is called surveillance.

The goal is:

- To monitor for changes
- To detect any progression early
- To intervene if needed

This approach provides safety and reassurance.

How It Is Managed

Management focuses on:

- Controlling acid reflux
- Using medications when needed
- Monitoring over time

If more advanced changes are detected, specific treatments may be used to remove or treat abnormal tissue.

Keeping a Balanced Perspective

It is natural to feel concerned when you hear about this condition.

But remember:

- It is not cancer
- Most patients do well
- Monitoring provides safety
- Early detection allows effective treatment

Understanding brings confidence.

A Practical Way to Think About It

Instead of asking, “How worried should I be?” ask:

“How can I stay informed and follow my care plan properly?”

That is the best approach.

Barrett's Esophagus

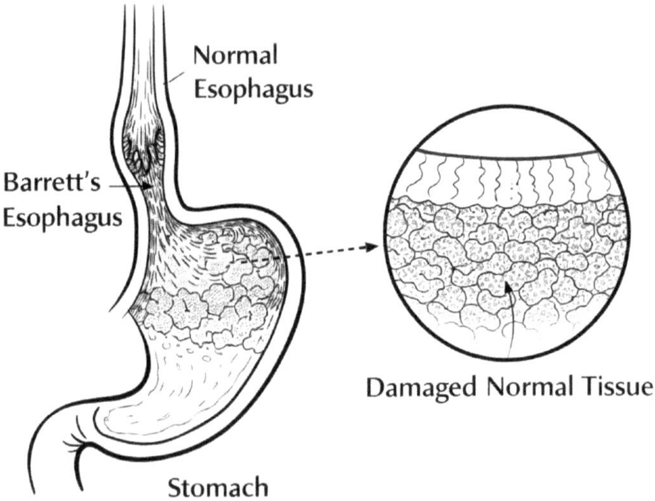

Serious Complication of Untreated Acid Reflux.

Increases Risk of Esophageal Cancer

Chapter Summary

Barrett's esophagus is a change in the lining of the esophagus due to long-term acid exposure. It increases the risk of certain complications, but the overall risk of cancer remains low for most patients.

Diagnosis requires endoscopy and biopsy, and regular follow-up helps ensure early detection of any changes.

Action Plan

If you have long-standing reflux:

- Discuss with your doctor whether evaluation is needed
- Follow recommended monitoring if diagnosed
- Continue managing reflux effectively

Stay informed, but remain calm.

Transition to Chapter 17

Reflux does not affect only the esophagus.

In the next chapter, we will explore how acid reflux can affect the throat, lungs, and teeth, often in subtle and unexpected ways.

Chapter 17

Reflux Affecting Other Organs

Why Reflux Is Not Just a Digestive Problem

Most people think of acid reflux as a problem limited to the chest or upper abdomen.

But in real clinical practice, it is often more than that.

Reflux can affect areas beyond the esophagus. In some patients, the main complaints are not heartburn at all. Instead, they come with throat symptoms, voice changes, cough, or even dental issues.

Because these symptoms are less obvious, the connection to reflux is often missed.

Understanding this broader picture helps you recognize symptoms early and avoid unnecessary confusion.

Throat Symptoms — Often Subtle but Persistent

Reflux can reach the upper part of the airway and irritate the throat.

Patients often describe:

- Frequent throat clearing
- A sensation of something stuck in the throat
- Mild irritation or dryness
- A persistent need to clear the throat

These symptoms are usually worse in the morning.

Many patients initially assume they are due to allergies or a mild infection.

Voice Changes and Hoarseness

The voice box is sensitive to irritation.

When exposed to acid:

- The voice may become hoarse
- Speaking may feel tiring
- The voice may sound rough or weak

People who use their voice frequently often notice this more clearly.

Chronic Cough — A Common but Missed Link

A persistent cough without clear cause is often evaluated repeatedly before reflux is considered.

This type of cough:

- Is usually dry

- May worsen at night
- Does not respond well to typical cough medications

Reflux may not be the only cause, but it can be an important contributor.

Effects on Breathing and Asthma

In some patients, reflux affects the airways.

It may:

- Worsen asthma symptoms
- Cause chest tightness
- Trigger episodes of breathlessness

This does not mean reflux is the only cause, but it can play a role and should be considered.

Laryngitis and Ongoing Throat Irritation

Repeated exposure to acid can inflame the voice box.

Patients may notice:

- Persistent throat discomfort
- Irritation that does not go away
- A constant need to clear the throat

These symptoms are often mild but long-lasting.

Dental Effects — An Overlooked Clue

Reflux can also affect the teeth.

When acid reaches the mouth repeatedly, it can:

- Erode the enamel
- Increase tooth sensitivity
- Lead to dental problems over time

Sometimes, dentists notice these changes before reflux is diagnosed.

Why These Symptoms Are Often Misunderstood

These symptoms are not specific to reflux.

They can also be caused by:

- Allergies
- Infections
- Smoking
- Environmental irritants

Reflux may be only one part of the picture.

This is why careful evaluation is important.

Recognizing the Pattern

If you experience these symptoms, ask yourself:

- Do they occur along with typical reflux symptoms?
- Are they worse at night or in the morning?
- Do they improve when reflux is treated?

Looking at the pattern helps guide diagnosis.

A Practical Perspective

Instead of focusing on one symptom, look at the overall pattern.

Reflux beyond the esophagus often presents as a combination of subtle, persistent symptoms rather than a single clear sign.

Chapter Summary

Acid reflux can affect areas beyond the esophagus, including the throat, voice, lungs, and teeth. Symptoms may include throat irritation, hoarseness, chronic cough, breathing problems, and dental changes.

These symptoms are often subtle and may have multiple causes, so careful evaluation is important.

Action Plan

If you have throat or breathing symptoms:

- Observe whether they relate to meals or nighttime
- Note any associated reflux symptoms
- Discuss these patterns with your doctor

Avoid assuming a single cause without proper evaluation.

Transition to Chapter 18

While many patients improve with lifestyle changes and medications, some may need additional treatment options.

In the next chapter, we will discuss when procedures or surgery may be considered and what they involve.

Chapter 18

When Procedures or Surgery May Help

Start With Reassurance

Let me begin with something very important.

Most people with acid reflux do not need surgery.

The majority improve with lifestyle changes and proper use of medication. That remains the foundation of treatment.

However, in some situations, additional options may be considered. Understanding these options will help you make informed and confident decisions if you ever reach that stage.

When Should Surgery Be Considered?

Surgery is not the first step. It is considered only in selected cases.

It may be appropriate when:

- Symptoms remain troublesome despite proper treatment
- Medications are required long term and the patient prefers an alternative
- Reflux is clearly confirmed through testing
- Complications such as significant inflammation are present

The most important point is this:

The diagnosis must be clear before considering surgery.

Fundoplication — The Most Established Procedure

The most commonly performed surgery for reflux is called **fundoplication**.

In simple terms:

- The upper part of the stomach is wrapped around the lower esophagus
- This strengthens the natural valve
- It reduces the backward flow of acid

This procedure is usually performed using minimally invasive techniques.

When done for the right reasons, it can provide significant relief.

What Results Can You Expect?

Many patients experience clear improvement after surgery.

However, it is important to have realistic expectations.

After surgery:

- Heartburn and regurgitation usually improve significantly
- Some patients may still need occasional medication
- A few may experience side effects such as difficulty swallowing or gas-related discomfort

Understanding this helps avoid disappointment.

Endoscopic Treatments — Less Invasive Options

There are newer procedures performed through an endoscope.

These aim to:

- Strengthen the lower esophageal sphincter
- Reduce reflux episodes

They are less invasive than surgery, but they may not be suitable for everyone.

Their effectiveness can vary depending on individual factors.

Bariatric Surgery — Addressing the Underlying Cause

In patients with significant obesity, weight is often a major contributor to reflux.

In such cases, bariatric surgery may be considered.

This approach:

- Promotes weight loss
- Reduces abdominal pressure
- Often improves reflux symptoms

It addresses the underlying cause rather than only the symptoms.

Why Careful Evaluation Is Essential

Before any procedure, a detailed evaluation is necessary.

This may include:

- Confirming reflux through testing
- Assessing esophageal function
- Reviewing overall health

Without proper evaluation, the outcome may not be satisfactory.

Balancing Benefits and Risks

Every procedure has both benefits and risks.

Surgery can provide long-term relief, but it also involves:

- Recovery time
- Possible side effects
- The need for follow-up care

The decision should always be thoughtful and individualized.

Take Your Time Before Deciding

Surgery is not an urgent decision in most cases.

It should be considered after:

- Trying appropriate medical treatment
- Confirming the diagnosis
- Understanding expected outcomes

Taking time to think leads to better choices.

A Practical Way to Think About It

Instead of asking, "Should I have surgery?" ask:

"Have I tried the right treatments, and is my diagnosis clearly confirmed?"

This approach helps guide the decision.

Chapter Summary

Most patients with GERD do not require surgery. However, in selected cases, procedures such as fundoplication, endoscopic treatments, or bariatric surgery may provide significant relief.

Careful evaluation and proper patient selection are essential for good outcomes.

Procedures and Surgeries for GERD

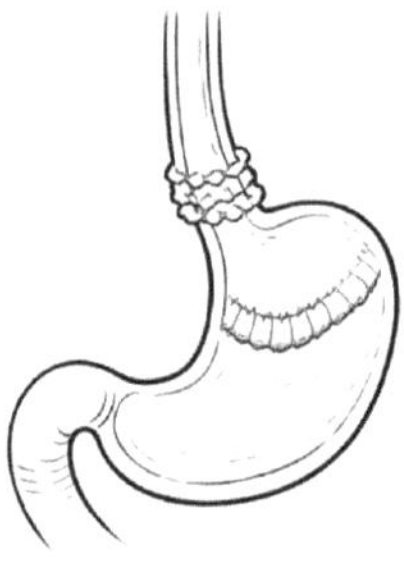

Fundoplication

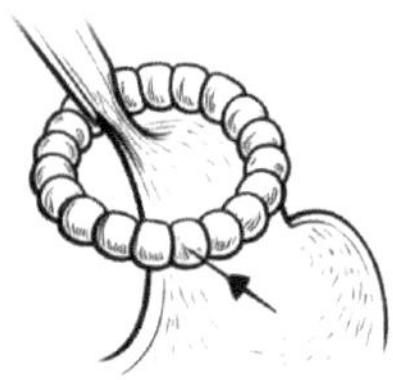

LINX Device

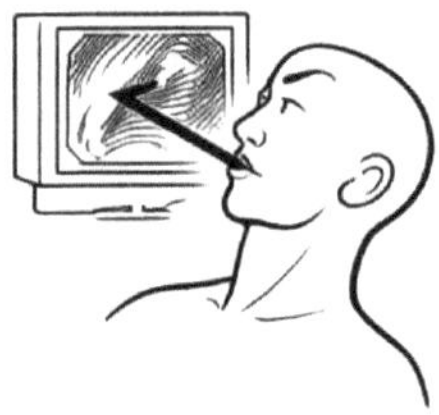

Endoscopic Therapy

Specialized Treatments When Lifestyle Changes and Medications Are Not Enough

Action Plan

If you are considering additional treatment:

- Confirm that your diagnosis is clear
- Understand the benefits and possible risks
- Discuss all options with your doctor

Make a thoughtful and informed decision.

Transition to Chapter 19

Reflux does not affect everyone in the same way.

In the next chapter, we will discuss special situations such as pregnancy, aging, and the use of multiple medications, where management needs to be more individualized.

Chapter 19
Special Situations

Why One Plan Does Not Fit Everyone

In real life, patients are different.

Some are young and otherwise healthy. Others are older, take multiple medications, or live with chronic health conditions. Some are pregnant. Some are dealing with excess weight.

In these situations, acid reflux does not always behave in the usual way.

Management needs to be thoughtful and individualized.

This chapter will help you understand how reflux is approached in these common, real-world situations.

Reflux During Pregnancy — Common and Usually Temporary

Reflux is very common during pregnancy.

This happens because:

- Hormonal changes relax the lower esophageal sphincter
- The growing uterus increases pressure inside the abdomen

Symptoms often become more noticeable as pregnancy progresses.

The reassuring part is this:

- Symptoms usually improve after delivery
- Simple lifestyle measures are often effective

Helpful steps include:

- Eating smaller meals
- Avoiding late-night eating
- Staying upright after meals

Medications may be used when necessary, but always under medical guidance.

Reflux in Older Adults — Often Less Typical

In older adults, reflux may not always present with classic heartburn.

Instead, patients may experience:

- Difficulty swallowing
- Unexplained weight loss
- Chest discomfort without clear burning

Older adults are also more likely to:

- Develop complications
- Take multiple medications
- Have other medical conditions

This makes careful evaluation and regular follow-up especially important.

Obesity — A Strong and Modifiable Risk Factor

Excess body weight is one of the most important contributors to reflux.

Increased abdominal pressure:

- Pushes the stomach upward
- Weakens the natural valve
- Increases frequency of symptoms

The encouraging part is this:

Even modest weight loss can lead to meaningful improvement.

Multiple Medications — An Overlooked Factor

Many patients take several medications for different conditions.

Some of these medicines can:

- Relax the lower esophageal sphincter
- Irritate the esophagus
- Worsen reflux symptoms

Examples include:

- Certain blood pressure medications
- Sedatives
- Some asthma medications
- Pain relievers such as NSAIDs

A careful review of medications with your doctor can be very helpful.

Reflux With Other Medical Conditions

Reflux often occurs along with other conditions such as:

- Diabetes
- Lung disease
- Heart conditions

These conditions can:

- Influence symptoms
- Affect treatment choices
- Require a more coordinated approach

Management in these cases should be tailored to the individual.

When Symptoms Do Not Follow the Usual Pattern

In special situations, symptoms may be:

- Less typical
- More persistent
- More difficult to treat

This is when a more detailed evaluation becomes important.

Personalizing Your Treatment Plan

The key message is simple.

Your treatment should reflect your situation.

This includes:

- Your age
- Your overall health
- Your medications
- Your lifestyle

A personalized approach leads to better results and safer care.

A Practical Way to Think About It

Instead of asking, “What is the standard treatment?” ask:

“What is the right treatment for me?”

That is the question that leads to better outcomes.

Chapter Summary

Acid reflux requires special consideration in situations such as pregnancy, older age, obesity, and in patients taking multiple medications or having other health conditions.

A personalized approach is essential for safe and effective management.

Action Plan

Reflect on your situation:

- Do you have any special factors such as pregnancy, weight concerns, or multiple medications?
- Have your medications been reviewed recently?
- Do your symptoms differ from typical reflux?

Discuss these points with your doctor to tailor your treatment plan.

Transition to Chapter 20

Even with good information, many patients are influenced by common myths and misunderstandings.

In the next chapter, we will clear these misconceptions so you can make more confident and informed decisions.

Chapter 20

Common Myths — Clearing Confusion

Why Misunderstanding Causes Unnecessary Suffering

In today's world, patients are surrounded by information.

Some of it is helpful. Much of it is confusing. And some of it quietly leads people in the wrong direction.

In my practice, I often see patients struggling not just with reflux, but with what they believe about it.

They avoid too many foods, fear helpful medications, or worry unnecessarily about serious disease.

Clearing these misconceptions is just as important as prescribing the right treatment.

Myth 1: "Heartburn Is Harmless, It Will Go Away"

Occasional heartburn is common and usually not serious.

But frequent or persistent symptoms should not be ignored.

If reflux becomes regular:

- It can affect sleep and daily life
- It may lead to complications over time

The right approach is awareness, not neglect.

Myth 2: "If I Do Not Feel Burning, It Cannot Be Reflux"

Many people believe reflux always causes a burning sensation.

This is not true.

Some patients have:

- Chronic cough
- Throat irritation
- Hoarseness
- Chest discomfort without burning

Reflux can present in different ways.

Relying only on heartburn may lead to missed diagnosis.

Myth 3: "Food Is the Only Cause"

Food plays a role, but it is not the only factor.

Reflux is influenced by:

- The function of the lower esophageal sphincter
- Body weight
- Meal timing
- Lifestyle habits

Focusing only on food can lead to unnecessary restrictions without solving the real problem.

Myth 4: "I Must Avoid Many Foods Completely"

Some patients come with a long list of foods they have stopped eating.

This often leads to frustration without real improvement.

The truth is:

- Not all foods affect everyone
- Personal triggers vary
- A balanced approach works better

You do not need extreme restriction. You need understanding.

Myth 5: "PPIs Are Dangerous and Should Be Avoided"

This is one of the most common concerns.

PPIs are effective medications.

When used appropriately:

- They relieve symptoms
- They help heal the esophagus

Like all medicines, they should be used thoughtfully. But avoiding them out of fear can lead to unnecessary discomfort.

Myth 6: "If Treatment Does Not Work, It Must Be Serious"

Many patients assume that persistent symptoms mean something serious.

In reality, symptoms may continue because:

- Medication is not used correctly
- Lifestyle factors are still present
- The diagnosis needs to be reassessed

Serious disease is not the most common explanation.

Myth 7: "Everyone With GERD Needs Surgery"

This is not true.

Most patients improve with:

- Lifestyle changes
- Proper use of medication

Surgery is reserved for selected cases.

Myth 8: "Once I Start Medication, I Will Need It Forever"

Many patients worry about this.

In reality:

- Some patients need short-term treatment
- Others may need longer-term use
- Many can reduce or stop medication over time

Treatment can be adjusted based on your progress.

Myth 9: "Reflux Is Only a Digestive Problem"

Reflux can affect:

- The throat
- The voice
- The lungs
- The teeth

Understanding this helps explain symptoms that may seem unrelated.

Replacing Myths With Clear Thinking

You do not need to remember every detail.

But you do need to think clearly.

When you replace myths with understanding:

- You reduce unnecessary fear
- You make better decisions
- You manage your condition more effectively

A Practical Way to Think About It

Instead of asking, "What have I heard about reflux?" ask:

"What do I understand about my own condition?"

That is what matters most.

Chapter Summary

Acid reflux is often surrounded by myths that lead to confusion and unnecessary worry. Misconceptions about symptoms, causes, and treatments can interfere with proper care.

Clear understanding allows you to manage your condition with confidence.

Action Plan

Reflect on your beliefs:

- Are you avoiding foods unnecessarily?
- Are you worried about medications without clear understanding?

- Are you assuming the worst about your symptoms?

Replace these concerns with informed, balanced decisions.

Transition to Chapter 21

Now that confusion has been cleared, it is time to bring everything together.

In the next chapter, we will create a simple and practical plan that you can follow step by step to take control of your reflux.

Chapter 21

Your Step-by-Step Plan to Take Control

Turning Knowledge Into Daily Action

You have now learned a great deal about acid reflux.

You understand what it is, why it happens, how it presents, and how it is treated.

But real improvement begins when you apply this knowledge in your daily life.

In this chapter, I will give you a clear, simple, and practical plan. This is the same structured approach I use with my patients. It is easy to follow and, more importantly, it works.

Step 1: Understand Your Symptoms Clearly

Everything begins with awareness.

Take a few days to observe:

- When your symptoms occur
- What seems to trigger them
- Whether they are worse after meals or at night

Do not rely on assumptions. Careful observation often reveals patterns that guide treatment.

Step 2: Make Practical Lifestyle Changes

Start with a few changes that have the greatest impact:

- Avoid lying down for at least 2 to 3 hours after meals
- Elevate the head of your bed
- Eat smaller, balanced meals
- Begin gradual weight reduction if needed

Do not try to change everything at once. Start small and stay consistent.

Step 3: Use Medicines Correctly

If medications are part of your treatment, use them properly.

- Take them at the correct time
- Take them regularly as advised
- Do not stop suddenly without guidance

Many patients improve simply by correcting how they take their medication.

Step 4: Identify Your Personal Triggers

Instead of avoiding many foods blindly, focus on your own triggers.

Ask yourself:

- Which foods clearly worsen my symptoms?
- Is it the type of food, the portion size, or the timing?

A personalized approach is more effective and easier to follow.

Step 5: Know When to Seek Medical Advice

Do not delay evaluation if:

- Symptoms persist despite treatment
- Warning signs appear
- Your symptoms change in pattern

Timely medical advice prevents complications and confusion.

Step 6: Monitor Your Progress

Improvement is usually gradual.

Track your progress:

- Are symptoms less frequent?
- Are they less severe?
- Is your sleep improving?

Small improvements are meaningful.

Step 7: Maintain Long-Term Control

Once you feel better, the goal is to stay better.

This includes:

- Continuing healthy habits
- Adjusting medication if needed
- Periodic reassessment

Think of this as ongoing care, not a temporary fix.

A Simple Framework to Remember

If you ever feel unsure, remember this sequence:

Understand ’! Adjust ’! Treat ’! Monitor ’! Maintain

This simple structure can guide you at every stage.

A Practical Way to Think About It

Instead of asking, “What more should I do?” ask:

“What is the next simple step I can take today?”

That is how progress happens.

Chapter Summary

Managing acid reflux requires a structured approach. Understanding symptoms, making practical lifestyle changes, using medications correctly, identifying personal triggers, and monitoring progress are essential steps.

Consistency and personalization are the keys to long-term success.

Action Plan

Start today with three simple steps:

- Observe your symptoms and triggers
- Make one meaningful lifestyle change
- Use your medication correctly if prescribed

Keep it simple and stay consistent.

Transition to Chapter 22

Taking control is the first step.

In the next chapter, we will focus on how to maintain that control over time and prevent symptoms from returning.

Chapter 22

Preventing Relapse and Staying in Control

Why Long-Term Thinking Changes Everything

Many patients feel much better after starting treatment.

Symptoms improve. Sleep becomes restful. Eating feels comfortable again.

Then, slowly and quietly, symptoms return.

This is very common.

Acid reflux is often not a one-time problem. It is a tendency that can return if earlier habits come back.

That is why the goal is not just relief. The goal is lasting control.

Build Habits That You Can Sustain

The most effective way to prevent relapse is not strict rules. It is simple habits that you can continue without difficulty.

Focus on:

- Regular meal timing
- Avoiding late-night eating
- Eating moderate portions
- Staying physically active

You do not need perfection. You need consistency.

Weight — A Long-Term Influence

Weight is not static. It changes over time.

Even a small increase in weight can bring symptoms back.

On the other hand:

- Modest weight loss improves symptoms
- Maintaining a stable weight helps prevent recurrence

Think of weight management as an ongoing effort, not a temporary goal.

Protect Your Sleep Routine

Good sleep habits remain essential.

Maintain:

- A gap of at least 2 to 3 hours between dinner and sleep

- Elevation of the head of your bed if needed
- A regular sleep schedule

Better sleep reduces symptoms, and better symptom control improves sleep.

Review Medication Periodically

Many patients continue medication without reassessment.

This is not always necessary.

It is important to:

- Review your need for medication periodically
- Adjust the dose when symptoms are controlled
- Avoid unnecessary long-term use

Some patients need ongoing treatment. Others can reduce or stop medication under guidance.

Recognize Early Signs of Relapse

Relapse usually does not happen suddenly.

It begins with small changes:

- Occasional return of symptoms
- Mild discomfort after certain meals
- Slight disturbance in sleep

Recognizing these early allows you to act before symptoms

become more frequent.

Stay Flexible, Not Rigid

One of the biggest challenges is balance.

You do not need strict, lifelong restrictions.

Instead:

- Be aware of your habits
- Allow occasional flexibility
- Return to good routines when symptoms reappear

This approach is practical and sustainable.

Maintain a Long-Term Partnership With Your Doctor

Your condition may change over time.

Regular follow-up helps:

- Adjust your treatment plan
- Monitor for complications when needed
- Maintain long-term control

Good care is always a partnership.

Confidence Comes With Experience

As you continue managing your condition, you will gain confidence.

You will begin to understand:

- What triggers your symptoms
- What helps you feel better
- How to respond early

This confidence is one of the most valuable outcomes.

A Practical Way to Think About It

Instead of asking, "Will my reflux come back?" ask:

"What can I do to keep it under control?"

That shift in thinking makes a difference.

Chapter Summary

Long-term control of acid reflux depends on consistent habits, weight management, good sleep routines, and periodic review of medication. Relapse is common but can be prevented with early recognition and timely action.

A balanced and sustainable approach leads to lasting success.

Action Plan

Focus on these steps:

- Maintain regular meal and sleep habits
- Monitor your weight

- Watch for early return of symptoms
- Review your treatment plan periodically

Consistency is more important than perfection.

Transition to Conclusion

You now have a complete understanding of acid reflux, from its causes to its long-term management.

In the final section, we will bring everything together and reinforce the key principles that will help you stay healthy and confident moving forward.

Conclusion

Take Control of Your Reflux

From Uncertainty to Understanding

When many patients first begin this journey, they are uncertain.

They are unsure about their symptoms. They are confused about food choices. They are concerned about medications and long-term risks.

If you pause for a moment and reflect, you will notice how far you have come.

You now understand your condition clearly.

And that understanding changes everything.

What Truly Matters — The Key Takeaways

If you remember only a few points from this book, let them be these:

- Acid reflux is common, but persistent symptoms should

not be ignored

- Symptoms can vary and are not always obvious
- Lifestyle changes are powerful and often essential
- Medicines are effective when used correctly
- Not all symptoms are due to reflux, so correct diagnosis matters
- Early attention helps prevent complications

These simple principles will guide you at every stage.

Avoid Fear. Choose Balance.

It is easy to feel overwhelmed by conflicting advice.

You may hear that certain foods must always be avoided. You may read about medication risks and feel uncertain. You may worry about serious disease.

Let me reassure you.

You do not need fear. You need balance.

Most people with reflux do not develop serious problems. At the same time, ignoring persistent symptoms is not wise.

The best approach lies between these two extremes.

Small Steps, Meaningful Change

You do not need dramatic changes to improve.

In fact, the most effective improvements often come from simple steps:

- Adjusting meal timing
- Improving sleep habits
- Maintaining a healthy weight
- Using medication correctly when needed

These small steps, when practiced consistently, lead to real and lasting improvement.

You Are in Control

One of the most rewarding moments in clinical practice is when a patient realizes this:

"I can manage this."

You begin to:

- Recognize your triggers
- Respond early to symptoms
- Make confident decisions

You are no longer reacting to your condition. You are managing it.

Work With Your Doctor, Not Alone

You do not have to manage this alone.

A thoughtful discussion with your doctor helps:

- Confirm your diagnosis

- Guide your treatment
- Adjust your plan over time

Good care is always a partnership.

A Final Thought

Acid reflux is not something you need to fear.

It is something you need to understand and manage.

With the knowledge you now have:

- You can reduce your symptoms
- You can improve your daily comfort
- You can protect your long-term health

Take one step at a time. Stay consistent. Stay informed.

And most importantly, take care of your health with confidence.

Chapter Summary

Acid reflux and GERD are common but manageable conditions. Understanding your symptoms, making practical lifestyle changes, using medications correctly, and seeking timely medical advice are the keys to effective control.

A calm, balanced, and consistent approach leads to long-term success.

Action Plan

Starting today:

- Identify one habit you can improve
- Use your medication correctly if prescribed
- Observe your symptoms calmly and clearly
- Plan a follow-up if needed

Small, consistent steps will lead to lasting results.

Appendix A

A Simple Daily Routine to Keep Acid Reflux Under Control

Morning — Start Your Day Calmly

- Begin your day with a glass of water
- Take your medication, if prescribed, **30–60 minutes before breakfast**
- Eat a light, balanced breakfast
- Eat slowly and avoid rushing

Midday — Maintain Balance

- Eat a moderate lunch, not too heavy
- Sit upright while eating
- Avoid lying down after meals

- Take a short walk if possible

Evening — Focus on Timing and Portion

- Eat dinner **at least 2–3 hours before bedtime**
- Keep dinner lighter than lunch
- Avoid overeating or second helpings

Night — Support Restful Sleep

- Do not lie down immediately after eating
- Elevate the head of your bed if needed
- Maintain a regular sleep routine

Key Takeaway

A steady, simple routine practiced daily is more effective than occasional strict efforts.

Appendix B

Common Trigger Foods — A Practical Guide

Foods That May Worsen Symptoms

Not everyone reacts the same way, but common triggers include:

- Fried and fatty foods
- Spicy foods
- Chocolate
- Coffee and tea
- Alcohol
- Carbonated drinks
- Citrus fruits
- Tomato-based foods

A Smarter Approach

Do not try to avoid everything.

Instead:

- Observe how your body responds
- Identify your personal triggers
- Reduce only what clearly affects you

Better Choices

- Prefer grilled, baked, or lightly cooked foods
- Eat smaller portions
- Choose mild, non-irritating foods
- Favor simple, home-cooked meals

Key Takeaway

Personalized choices work better than strict restrictions.

Appendix C

Medication Guide — Simple & Clear

Antacids

- Provide quick relief
- Short duration of action
- Best for occasional symptoms

H2 Blockers

- Moderate reduction of acid
- Useful for mild to moderate symptoms
- Helpful for nighttime symptoms

Proton Pump Inhibitors (PPIs)

- Most effective for frequent symptoms
- Help heal the esophagus
- Must be taken **before meals** for best results

Important Reminders

- Take medications at the correct time
- Do not skip doses
- Do not stop suddenly without guidance
- Review long-term use periodically with your doctor

Key Takeaway

Correct use of medication is essential for good results.

Appendix D

When to Seek Medical Help

Seek medical attention promptly if you experience:

- Difficulty swallowing
- Pain while swallowing
- Vomiting blood or material that looks like coffee grounds
- Black, tarry stools
- Unexplained weight loss
- Persistent vomiting
- Chest pain with exertion or shortness of breath

Key Takeaway

Do not delay evaluation when warning signs are present.

Appendix E

Your Two-Week Food and Symptom Diary

Use this simple format:

Day	What I Ate & When	Symptoms	Possible Trigger
Day 1	Dinner at 8 PM	Heartburn at 10 PM	Heavy meal
Day 2			

How to Use This Diary

- Record daily for 1–2 weeks
- Be honest and consistent
- Look for patterns, not isolated events

Key Takeaway

Patterns provide clarity and guide better decisions.

Appendix F

Your Personal Acid Reflux Control Plan

My Main Symptoms

My Common Triggers

My Daily Habits to Improve

My Medication Plan

My Follow-Up Plan

Key Takeaway

When you write your plan clearly, you are more likely to follow it and succeed.

Thank You and Please Review the Book

Thank you for taking the time to read this book. I sincerely hope it has helped you understand your health a little more clearly and has given you practical, everyday steps you can follow with confidence. If you found this book helpful, **I would truly appreciate it if you could leave a brief and honest review.** Even a few lines sharing your experience can make a meaningful difference. Your feedback helps other readers find reliable, trustworthy health information and supports them in making better decisions for themselves and their families.

Warm regards,

Dr Prabhat Das

Continue your Healthcare Journey

Good health is a journey, not a single step. It is not achieved in one day or with one book. That is why I created the "Better Health with Dr Das" series, with each book addressing a different common condition. If you would like easy, practical guidance on other everyday health concerns, you may wish to explore the rest of books in this series.

Books in this series:

- Better Health starts Here: A Doctor's Guide to Staying Healthy After 40
- A Doctor's Easy Guide to Understanding & Managing OBESITY
- Doctor, What DIET Is Best for Me?
- Doctor, Why Can't I Lose Weight? A Doctor's Guide to safe & Sustainable Weight Loss)
- A Doctor's Easy Guide to GLP-1 for Obesity
- A Doctor's Easy Guide to Understanding &

Managing HIGH BLOOD PRESSURE

- A Doctor's Guide to Living Well With DIABETES
- A Doctor's Guide to Understanding & Managing THYROID DISEASES
- A Doctor's Guide to Understanding & Managing HIGH CHOLESTEROL
- A Doctor's Practical Guide to HEART HEALTH After 40: How to Protect Your Heart & Live Longer
- A Doctor's Guide to Healing & Reversing FATTY LIVER DISEASE: Simple, Natural & Science-Based Steps to Reduce Liver Fat and Prevent Complications
- Control Your ACID REFLUX, HEARTBURN & GERD: A Doctor's Practical Guide that Works
- Live Comfortably with IRRITABLE BOWEL SYNDROME: A Doctor's Practical Guide to Understanding & Managing IBS
- A Doctor's Practical Guide to Understanding & Managing GALLBLADDER STONES & OTHER PROBLEMS
- Take Control of COPD: A Doctor's Practical Guide to Better Breathing
- Living Better Life with ASTHMA: A Doctor's Practical Guide to Asthma Control
- SLEEP APNEA & SNORING: A Doctor's Practical Guide to Better Sleep & Better Health

- KIDNEY STONES: A Doctor's Practical Guide to Prevention & Care
- Protect Your KIDNEYS: A Doctor's Practical Guide to Kidney Health & Prevention
- PROSTATE HEALTH After 40: A Doctor's Practical Guide to Early Detection & Care
- ARTHRITIS: A Doctor's Practical Guide to Pain Control & Mobility
- A Doctor's Practical Guide to Fixing BACK PAIN Step by Step
- A Doctor's Practical Guide to Understanding & Managing GOUT & URIC ACID and Preventing Complications
- HEALTHY SKIN & COMMON SKIN PROBLEMS: A Doctor's Practical Guide to Skin Care
- DEMENTIA & MEMORY LOSS: A Doctor's Practical Guide to Prevention & Management
- Doctor, Why Am I TIRED All The Time? Fixing Fatigue & Getting Your Energy Back

Printed by Libri Plureos GmbH in Hamburg,
Germany

9 781971 672274